I dedicate this book to my wonderful children,
Alexandra and Adam, and to Phil, the best husband
and partner imaginable. You have given me the
most rewarding, the most validating, the ultimate
experience of life—motherhood.

contents

acknowledgments

"What is your dream?" I was asked. That was the first question my publicist, Harris Shepard, posed to me. I answered, "To help people everywhere in the world live happier, healthier lives." Without Harris, this book would never have happened. Through him, I met Paddy Calistro McAuley, my writing partner, whose help in putting my voice into words was invaluable and beyond words. I'm thankful, too, for the help of her husband, Scott McAuley, and assistant Lindsay Hagans.

Indebted I am to Barbara Lowenstein, literary agent extraordinaire, who made the book a reality. I am eternally grateful, as well, to Megan Newman, publisher at Avery, whose vision and enthusiasm for the concept brought *Body After Baby* to fruition, and to my editor, Lucia Watson, and Claire Vaccaro, the art director who shaped the form and look of these pages. And speaking of art, kudos and thanks to Peter Young, who illustrated *Body After Baby,* and to Cathy Guisewite for introducing him to me and our project.

I am indebted, too, to my friend Kathy Smith for her insight and helpful guidance, and I am grateful for the wonderful foreword she contributed. Many thanks, also, to the experts whose words are included in these pages—they are health professionals whom I am honored to call friends: Cindy Moskovic, MSW; Liliana Sloninsky, M.D.; W. Kip Johnson, M.D.; Linda Steele, Ph.D.; Margaret England,

M.D.; Susan Bowerman, M.S., R.D.; Rick Barke; Alicia Trocker, M.S., R.D.; Michael Tabak, M.D.; and Shari Kahane, M.D., R.N. My gratitude goes, too, to Cheri Lowre, M.D.; Sheri Barke, M.S., R.D.; and Sheila King, M.S., for validating the spirit of this book.

Thanks to my staff at NutriFit, for their support and patience: Keegan Sheridan, Megan McElwee, Kris Reid, Deirdra Martinez, Gretchen Zegarra, Nelva Ventura and the Reveco family, Hugo, Mariana, Matias, and Millaray (who at the age of one week became the model baby for the illustrations). To Dian Thomas, Jane Mannfolk, Tania Cobb, and Dawn Feldman Mills, colleagues and clients, this includes you! Thank you, Stan McClurkin-Birge, for conquering the software challenges of the recipe section of this book.

I'm particularly grateful to the staff at Harris Shepard Public Relations, and public relations agents Erin Jundef, Jess Rodriguez, Dana Sarbeck, Meredith Greene, and Kerry Hopkins, television producer Gerri Shaftel, and writers Debbie Emery and Caroline Schaffer for helping make me and NutriFit known to many.

Were it not for the help of friends and trainers Phil Landman, Stephanie McCusker, Rick Barke, Mak Takano, and Jon Jon Park, I would not have been able to maintain my equanimity—so thanks, guys, for helping me stay sane and fit.

When it comes to patronage, I'm a real fan of my local grocery store, where I've come to be known for my prodigious food purchases and recycled bags. To Gabriel Garcia, June Nonnette, Norma Matsuguma, Bob Tong, and Romero Profirio, thanks for your support and for making my life easier.

Finally, to all the *Body After Baby* moms who shared their stories, thank you for being so open and receptive, and for allowing me to bring your experience to others.

foreword by kathy smith

YOU'VE PROBABLY SEEN Jackie Keller on television talking about healthy nutrition. Or maybe you've read about her in newspapers and magazines. Jackie is the nutrition coach to some of Hollywood's biggest stars. And, she has turned around the lives of thousands of women whose names aren't as well known, but whose concerns are just as important to her.

I met Jackie right after I had my second baby, at a time when I was the working mother of two, with exercise videos to produce, books to write, and no time to cook. During those hectic years, a steady diet of Jackie's healthy gourmet food-delivery service, NutriFit, was the wisest gift I ever gave myself. Not only did it simplify my life, it brought me into contact with this talented kindred spirit. Now, after years of enjoying her wonderful food, and countless hours spent discussing the benefits of healthy eating and exercise, I can say this from experience: Jackie's a culinary master, and a genuine nutritional guru. I'm so excited that she's finally sharing her wisdom—and those fabulous recipes—with a wider audience in *Body After Baby*.

What I love about Jackie is that she is absolutely straightforward and smart. And what I love about her *Body After Baby* program is the very same thing: it's clear, concise, and, like Jackie, very, very smart. After working with many new moms, Jackie realized that mothers with new babies yearn for three things: they want more energy, they want sounder sleep, and they want their bodies back. In response to their needs—*your* needs—Jackie has developed nutritious ways to accomplish all three. No gimmicks, just good, wholesome food loaded with nutrients, coupled with a sound exercise program.

Reading her book, I was struck by how perfectly Jackie's understanding of the new mom's predicament fit my own experience. Sixteen years ago, pregnant and filming my *Pregnancy Workout,* I learned firsthand how anxious women are about their bodies during those otherwise joyous months. And, sure enough, after giving birth, I was faced with exactly the issues Jackie identifies. I couldn't wait to get back into the jeans I'd worn prepregnancy. I was eager to get back to my highly active lifestyle, but still low on energy. And oh, how I wanted a good night's sleep! Not to mention that, after forty weeks of pregnancy, I really wanted to feel sexy again. Jackie's solutions to these universal problems are a wonderful blend of sensitivity, wisdom, and practical know-how.

As a working mom with two great kids of her own, Jackie understands that you don't want to take time away from your baby and your family. And so, she shows you how to select nutrient-rich foods that are quick and easy to prepare. She also shows you how to get a complete workout by exercising for brief intervals throughout the day—ten minutes here, ten minutes there—whenever you have an extra moment. There's always time to move in her program, and it never has to be drudgery.

And she shows you why the period right after your baby arrives is a critical time—the *ideal* time—to get back in shape, for several reasons. First, your body has a memory. After being stretched and strained, it wants to get back to its prepregnancy state. Second, your hormones are telling your body to lose weight, so there is never a better time to adopt a sensible nutrition and exercise program. Third, now that you have created one new life, it's the perfect time to give your own life a healthy, new start. The fact is, when you replenish yourself and feel good about it, you can nourish everyone around you. The joyous, patient, and loving being that is *you* comes through loud and clear. That's the best example you can set for your family.

Take it from me, we mothers *are* role models. Our kids learn from us every minute. When you favor nutritious foods, good nutrition becomes your child's expectation. When you choose to go for a walk instead of watching television, your child gets the movement message. My girls and I have been on walks together since *before* they could walk—when they were still in packs on their daddy's and my backs. Later, when they were old enough for bikes, we rode together. And we still do; we're an active bunch. I didn't think about it then, but now I give myself credit for being a positive role model. Do the same for your kids and you'll discover how good it feels, on so many levels.

In *Body After Baby*, Jackie Keller makes good nutrition and healthy exercise the kinds of habits you'll *want* to get into. She shows you how to get back into shape sensibly—at your own pace—after your baby is born. You'll feel energized, you'll love the food, and you'll lose weight. Your body will come back better than ever, and so will your self-confidence. But *Body After Baby* is not a crash diet that has you working out for hours every day till you drop the pounds. It's all based on sound nutritional information, good planning, regular exercise, and, above all, consistency. Throughout this book, Jackie's message is that you've got to take care of yourself so you can take good care of your baby. Her *Body After Baby* program makes perfect sense. It's a great way to really take care of yourself when you need it most—right now!

you're ready for
body after baby

It's all about desire:

Your desire for a child.

Your desire for energy, for health, for renewed strength.

Your desire to look your best, to feel positive about your body again.

Your desire to recapture your prepregnancy self.

It's what brought you to this book.

You're ready for *Body After Baby*.

You've spent the last forty weeks creating perfection, and every time you look into your baby's eyes or hold those little hands you are reminded that every extra pound you gained was worth it. Now, though your hormones are raging, you're exhausted, and you're overwhelmed—you're the happiest you've ever been. When you look in the mirror, you know you're ready to fulfill your other desires. You want your body back.

The good news is that in the same way nature helped you add weight to nurture the new life that was growing inside of you, nature is going to help you shed the pounds that you don't need anymore. Everything in your body is ready to support your effort to get back into shape. That's why the *Body After Baby* plan works so well—it is structured to meet to your body's needs right now. If you follow the plan, you'll see up to twenty pounds of the weight you gained during pregnancy disappear in thirty days and you won't feel that overwhelming hunger or fatigue that's associated with "diets." The meals I've designed for you are filled with Super Fuel foods, nutrient-rich foods that give your body the energy it needs exactly when you need it. Plus, Super Fuel foods will help you sleep more soundly, help you to maintain your even temperament and your clear head, and provide the energy you need to take care of your newly expanded family. And a big plus, eating a healthy and balanced menu of Super Fuel foods every day will help your body drop its extra weight. You'll see the positive results—you'll be amazed at how dramatically your body can change in thirty days.

It Really Works

When I founded NutriFit—L.A.'s premier gourmet meal service that prepares and delivers nutritious gourmet meals, individualized to the client's specific needs—I recognized an immediate need: Most moms have careers that demand they're back to the office, back to the courtroom, back to the operating room, back to the classroom, back to the boardroom, or back on the set of the next film in just a few short months. And all new moms, whether they are working outside the home or at home, are anxious to get their energy back so they can tend to their new baby's needs, sleep better, and get back to their prepregnancy weight. Like you, the women I meet through NutriFit are determined to lose the baby weight and feel good about themselves again. And they want to do it as soon as possible. So I created the *Body After Baby* plan: three meals a day, three snacks, all nutrient-rich and delicious. The plan is designed to help you and every postpartum mom shed the weight and gain energy—fast.

Time and again, I've seen the *Body After Baby* plan provide amazing results. Uma Thurman followed my plan and went from gaining nearly fifty-eight pounds during her pregnancy to achieving the svelte, killer body she showed off in the films *Kill Bill: Vol. 1* and *Vol. 2*. When she first came to me, her second baby was three months old and Uma had already lost about thirty-five pounds. But those last twenty pounds weren't coming off. She was exhausted and discouraged. Her director Quentin Tarantino was a client at NutriFit, the company I cofounded with my husband, Phil, in 1987. NutriFit provided food for the entire *Kill Bill* cast—Uma, Lucy Liu, Vivica A. Fox, Daryl Hannah, David Carradine, and, of course, Quentin himself. When he realized Uma needed some help, Quentin sent her to me for a special postpregnancy weight-loss program. The plan I designed for Uma helped her lose the remaining postpartum weight plus a few extra pounds. Uma was happy, Quentin was happy, and I think I may have been the happiest of all. But the best part is that the food plan Uma and many of my other clients were following will work for you, too, and you can follow it at home.

Body After Baby has helped plenty of other Hollywood moms slim down, too; my client list includes Uma, Angelina Jolie, Josie Bissett, Marcia Gaye Harden, Susan Sarandon, Tia Carrere, Lisa Rinna, Shamicka Lawrence (Mrs. Martin Lawrence), Marie Osmond (who has eight children, five of them adopted), and Ryan Haddon. Some came to me immediately after their babies were born, others waited years. And they all came to me because they wanted the same thing you do: improved stamina, increased energy, and weight loss. But they each had their own challenges, which points out one very important fact: no matter what your body type, how much weight you have gained during your pregnancy, how old you are, or how long it has been since your child was born, you can get back to a healthy weight. You can achieve exactly what you desire on the *Body After Baby* plan, while eating delicious meals that are packed with high-powered nutrition and following its safe, simple movement program.

Body After Baby is for all new moms, moms just like you, moms who all have individual needs, moms like my client Sammie who came to me after she had gained twenty-nine pounds during her pregnancy. I loved watching Sammie stand on the scale the day her baby turned four weeks old and seeing the joy she felt when she realized she'd lost thirty-one pounds. She started the plan the day she got home from the hospital and followed it faithfully. Here's what she told me: "It was so easy because I knew exactly what to eat, how to work exercise into my day, and how to shop for healthy food. I always had things to eat available, so I didn't reach for junk food—and when I wanted a snack, I knew what to have that was delicious and good for me."

It was a similar story for Anne, who came to me a few weeks after she had her baby. She had put on forty-five pounds during her pregnancy and had already lost about eleven pounds just in baby weight (baby was 7.2 pounds, placenta two pounds and amniotic fluid two pounds) when she started the plan. By carefully following the plan, in four weeks she had lost another eighteen pounds, twenty-nine pounds in all. She told me afterward: "The weight loss was terrific. But the best part was that my energy level was awesome, almost immediately. Before I started *Body After Baby* I felt so drained all the time. After a few days on the program I realized that I was buzzing around doing everything I wanted to do, plus I was sleeping better—whenever my baby let me sleep, that is."

The basis of the eating plan is well-chosen calories from foods rich in nutrients and phytochemicals, which will help you feel better and drop excess weight after your baby is born. There's absolutely no need to give up delicious-tasting foods. And there's no reason to go hungry. When you are eating nutrient-rich food, you'll feel full on fewer calories. The best part is that you'll enjoy delicious meals on my plan. So good that you won't believe they actually *help* you lose weight. You'll feel satisfied because the foods are rich in flavor. Plus, many of the foods you've thought were "bad" for you when you're trying to cut carbs, control fat, or count calories on various "diets" are actually *good* for you. For instance, both avocados and nuts—two foods that have been taboo on most weight-loss diets—are actually very rich in nutrients and provide essential energy on the *Body After Baby* plan. And for all you chocolate fans out there, a little dark chocolate before bed may help you sleep and provides beneficial plant chemicals—so you can look forward to having a little chocolate if you want it. Not what you expect to hear when the subject is healthy eating, right? But it's proven to be true, and you'll see that it works.

The secret to losing weight *while* gaining energy is Super Fuel foods—foods that have nutritious calories, which provide the energy you need to get the most out of your day. My meal plans and recipes are full of these healthful foods. Another secret is being sure to eat *enough* food—on my plan you'll enjoy three mouthwatering meals a day and three snacks. You need to eat enough food to be sure you get a healthy mix of vitamins and minerals, and help your body get back into balance. The plan is designed for nursing moms, but if you're bottle-feeding your little one, I provide alternatives that will keep your weight loss steady and your energy level high.

The *Body After Baby* plan isn't an extreme crash diet; it is based on proven principles of sound nutrition—principles that I want you to understand. When you understand the nutrition concepts behind the plan, it will be easier for you to make wise choices as you plan what you and your family are going to eat—now and in the future.

Making Yourself a Priority

Margo, one of my *Body After Baby* moms, called me in a panic just a few days after her baby was born. She was, by her own admission, a nervous mom. She worried about everything, but especially about breast-feeding, since her infant, Catharina, was exhibiting symptoms of discomfort after each nursing session. After several conversations, I understood the major reason Margo was worried. She asked for and accepted virtually everyone's advice—that of her housekeeper, her hairdresser, and her friends. Every time she asked for someone's advice, she modified her diet and, before long, her food choices were inconsistent, inadequate, and very limited. She was nutritionally starving her baby and herself and she didn't realize it. After she gave birth, I worked with her right away to incorporate more healthy vegetables and grains into her diet—she had taken them out for fear that they were making her nursing baby "sick and gassy." As she began to eat better, her own mood stabilized and her nerves quieted, and that helped her child immediately. As the whole breast-feeding experience improved, so did her baby's gas and Margo's disposition.

Margo was trying so hard to be a good mom and listen to everyone else, that both she and her baby were suffering. When your baby arrives, it's only natural to make your child your first priority. It's the unusual woman who makes a concerted effort to nurture herself during those wonderful but complicated months after giving birth. In fact, many women feel guilty about their desire to take care of

balanced nutrition is essential

MOTHERHOOD taxes the body, altering hormonal levels, emotional states, and sleep-wake cycles. In addition, in the early postpartum period, many mothers are temporarily anemic, due to blood loss during the delivery. Therefore, a well-balanced, iron-rich diet is preferable. While some women may feel the need to rigorously diet, this is not advisable. On the other end of the spectrum, while "fast food" may be a tempting, time-efficient alternative, this option is also not a wise choice. Staying with the basics— a well-balanced diet—will help both the breast-feeding and non-breast-feeding mother to optimize her own health and, both directly and indirectly, the health of her infant.

—MICHAEL TABAK, M.D.
Neonatologist, Kaiser Permanente Hospital and
Medical Center, Woodland Hills, California

themselves—they feel it takes away precious time from their child or children. But it's essential to take care of yourself. You can't make your best effort as a mother if you don't. It's like those safety instructions on airplanes that tell you to put your oxygen mask on first and then help your child—they make sense, don't they? Taking good care of yourself every day makes sense because you need to feel strong and healthy in order to raise a strong and healthy child. My eating and exercise plans provide the tools—you *will* be stronger from the very first day.

When I talk to new mothers, I find that although they are extremely focused, there are two main things they yearn for. Here's what they tell me:

1. **"I want enough energy to get through each day."** Your body is recovering from birth, hormones are going wild, and your sleep patterns are totally confused. Considering that a mom who breast-feeds burns about 500 to 600 extra calories daily (and moms who nurse multiple infants burn even more), it's no wonder you're dragging, especially if the food you're eating is not supernutritious. Plus you've got to sleep soundly, when you *do* sleep, and the *Body After Baby* plan will make that possible. The foods you eat will help calm you and ready your body for sound, satisfying sleep.

2. **"I want my body back."** You've spent nine months barely seeing your toes. You've had dreams about wearing a belt. You couldn't wait for the baby to be born so you'd have your body back, but now you're carrying extra weight, and that means you've got some extra fat, plus less muscle tone than you had before you were pregnant. And you've got even less time to devote to exercise. Don't worry. Relief is on its way.

It's imperative that you make it a priority to take care of your health during this transitional time, both for yourself and for your baby. I know what's possible, and together we can achieve it.

GET INTO THE MOVEMENT MODE

The *Body After Baby* plan has a twofold focus: food *and* physical activity. Doctors with whom I consult on a regular basis agree that gentle activity is perfectly safe postpartum, so you can begin easy movements as soon as possible after delivery. I'll show you ways to integrate exercise into your regular activities, simple ways to work your muscles and to feel more energetic. Whether you're working or staying at home with your child, the exercise portion of the *Body After Baby* plan provides short, structured workouts that will be supereffective. I'll illustrate the exercises you need to reshape your temporarily expanded body—movements that will be the fun and easy part of the plan. Adopting a long-term movement mind-set can be a bigger challenge. If you are determined to lose your baby weight, you'll see that regular exercise speeds the process *and* it provides you with the strength that you forgot you had! That's a big incentive to get moving.

Just as I tell my clients on a daily basis, it's important to understand that activity is not only a positive for you, but for your baby, too. I'm a firm believer that babies learn from their mothers at the earliest ages. If you make regular exercise an integral part of your day, your children will learn by example, and the earlier you start, the better. In chapter 7, I give you exercises that you can do with your baby. When a baby looks forward to doing mom-and-baby exercises, movement becomes a reward. Infants love the attention and movement of these exercises, and they'll learn quickly that exercise is something to look forward to. If you reinforce that with smiles, laughter, and joy, being active becomes an easy habit for your child to adopt and be enthusiastic about. And you'll enjoy the process, too—the quality time you'll have with your baby will be extraordinary.

LOSE THAT EXCESS WEIGHT NOW!

It's a fact: women who attend to their own nutrition and exercise needs immediately after the birth of a child have renewed energy, are healthier, and, yes, get back into shape faster. An important study published in *Obesity Research* reported that women who retained excess weight at the end of the first year postpartum were more likely to be overweight fifteen years later. My *Body After Baby* plan is designed to make sure that you are not overweight years from now. It's a plan that gets the weight off and keeps it off. Once you develop a pattern of healthy eating and get into an active lifestyle, you will simply eat wholesome foods in appropriate proportions and stay active.

The *Body After Baby* plan will help you lose weight whether you start immediately after delivery or when your baby is older. But if you start as soon as your baby is born you will have two distinct advantages: (1) During the immediate postpartum period, your hormones are working hard to help your body shed the fat you've accumulated during pregnancy. (2) You're getting all the nutrients you need for successfully breast-feeding your child and to keep you strong and healthy (whether you're breast-feeding or not) during the busy time ahead.

Because the foods you eat will help you sleep more soundly and help you feel more energetic, you'll have an easier time getting through the first several weeks after you bring your baby home. If you let some time pass after delivery before you begin, your weight loss may be slower, depending on how long you wait. But you will immediately benefit from the complete nutrition the *Body After Baby* meal plans provide, so there is never a time that is "too late" to start.

why lose weight now?

Two things are critical after a woman delivers her baby: that the child is nurtured and the mother feels content. When the new mother is happy, bonding with her baby is a naturally pleasurable experience. For a woman to have a positive postpartum experience, high self-esteem is essential. A new mother wouldn't think of not taking care of her child, but she must be as determined about taking care of herself. A big part of that is eating well and exercising so she can attain a healthy level of fitness as soon as possible. When a new mother can get close to her prepregnancy weight and activity level through appropriate food and exercise, she will be happier and healthier and will adapt well to her new role in life. The result? Happy mother, happy baby.

—LILIANA SLONINSKY, M.D.
Pediatric Hematologist, Assistant Clinical Professor,
UCLA Tri-Campus Pediatric Residency Program, Cedars-Sinai Medical Center, Mattel Children's Hospital at UCLA, Los Angeles County–Olive View Medical Center

ESTABLISHING YOUR GOAL

Now is the best time to reach a healthy weight, but many of my clients are confused about how to determine that goal. I always suggest using the body mass index. You probably know it by its acronym, BMI, which calculates your approximate percentage of body fat, based on your height and weight. Although the BMI isn't perfect (it doesn't account for additional muscle weight on very muscular people), it's an accepted method of finding your best weight, one that has stood the test of time and science. Use the BMI chart on page 347 to determine the optimal weight range for your height. Since BMI is used to calculate the approximate percentage of fat in your body, you probably are curious to know what your BMI is today. You can calculate your BMI body fat percentage easily with this formula:

$$\frac{\text{weight in pounds}}{(\text{height in inches}) \times (\text{height in inches})} \times 703 = \text{BMI}$$

A BMI range under 25 percent is desirable. Between 25 percent and 29.9 percent is overweight, and over 30 percent can be dangerous to your health. Don't worry if you are in higher ranges right now—by sticking to the *Body After Baby* plan, you'll lower your BMI percentage as your weight drops off.

WHAT HAPPENS TO YOUR BODY AFTER YOU DELIVER YOUR BABY?

A great deal happens the minute your baby is born. First, you may lose about nine to fifteen pounds the very first day—anywhere from six to ten pounds of baby, one to two pounds of placenta, and two to three pounds of amniotic fluid. No wonder you're exhausted the first few days! The rest of the weight gain you experienced is stored fat, which your body begins to use for energy. Nature provides that stored fat so you'll have the additional calories your body needs while breast-feeding.

Your metabolism will most likely increase as soon as you begin to nurse, since it takes a great deal of energy to manufacture breast milk. Breast-feeding requires up to an additional 500 to 600 calories per day, depending on how much your baby consumes.

The other amazing thing that happens is that your hormones react in a way that is unique to the postpartum period in a woman's life. At delivery, two hormones that we don't hear much about, leptin and serotonin, work together to put your body in a weight-loss mode. While no one's quite sure how leptin works, we do know that leptin levels stay elevated in your blood throughout your pregnancy. Leptin is released by fat tissue and signals the brain to limit fat intake. At delivery, leptin levels drop, which allows you to reset your body's "set point" to a prepregnancy level. Your metabolism continues working at a fast pace, burning more calories than usual to give you extra energy (*unless* you skip meals, which causes your metabolism to slow down!). The serotonin that your brain releases in response to the increased metabolism actively works to control your energy balance and helps keep your appetite in check. So as long as you're eating a healthy, lower-fat diet, your body will stay in this hormone-induced weight-loss mode. That's why I urge you to start the *Body After Baby* plan as soon after your delivery as you can.

Even though all those hormones are working to help you slim down, once the baby arrives, gravity can sometimes make your tummy look pretty saggy. All that stretched-out skin and muscle can't bounce back immediately, but it will! I know it might be discouraging right now, but don't despair—it won't be that way for long. If you are breast-feeding, your uterus contracts in response to nursing and will rather quickly return to its original size. Many women feel the contractions and liken them to menstrual cramps, but every "cramp" is actually doing good things to reduce the size of your uterus and, in turn, your tummy. Breast-feeding or not, you'll be amazed at how effective the *Body After Baby* movements are; your stomach muscles will respond and you'll see results very quickly.

Postpartum moms can develop thyroid problems such as decreased thyroid function or an inflammation of the thyroid gland (thyroiditis). That can slow down your metabolism, which can result in fatigue and difficulty losing weight. Signs of decreased thyroid function are numerous, but include hair loss and a body temperature lower than 98.6°F, so if you have difficulty losing weight on the *Body After Baby* plan and have these symptoms, check with your health-care professional.

OFF-TO-WORK MOMS

Of all my clients, I think Monica dreaded going back to work the most. Even though she was getting a little stir-crazy and restless with no other adults to talk to for most of the day, she hated the thought of leaving her wonderful baby. She had three months of maternity leave, but at the end of the second month, duty called. She knew that if she was going to keep her great position with the County of Los Angeles, a job she had always enjoyed, she would have to adopt a working-mom mind-set. She started planning. The first thing she realized was that with fifteen postpartum pounds still lingering, her work clothes weren't going to fit comfortably. She called NutriFit, and we put her on the *Body After Baby* plan. She loved the structure of three meals and three snacks a day. It made sense to her. And even though she had never been into exercise before, the *Body After Baby* movements were easy to incorporate into her day. She loved doing the mom-and-baby exercises, and since she was already taking her child for walks in the stroller she just upped the pace a bit. It took Monica four weeks to lose the last fifteen pounds, and she was thrilled to fit into her clothes again. She felt great about her accomplishment. Monica went back into the business world confident, fit, energized, and, best of all, secure in a new routine of healthy eating and exercise.

Going back to work can be difficult for any new mother. Like Monica, you may hate the thought of leaving your little one, no matter how trusted and experienced your chosen child-care provider is. You may feel alone and cheated out of time with your baby. Sometimes depression sets in. But the fact is, most new mothers who have jobs go back to work outside the home. And if you're one of those working moms, you will tend to lose more weight than other moms who stay at home. The reasons are well defined: structure and mental stimulation. Moms who work have a busy day, with specific times for eating the midday meal and specific break time for snacks. Because you are concentrating on your work, you are less likely to think about eating. When you get home, your family becomes the focus, so you're busy managing the home front. *Body After Baby* meals are designed to be appealing to the entire family, making planning and cooking easier. Your whole family will enjoy the foods, so you won't feel singled out for being on a diet. And the lunches and snacks adapt perfectly for brown bagging.

STAY-AT-HOME MOMS

From the time she was sixteen, Emily had always worked, but now, at thirty-one, she had interrupted her successful banking career to have her daughter, Megan, and she and her husband decided she would stay at home with the baby. It was great for the first several weeks, especially since John took two weeks of family leave and her parents had flown in from Minnesota to help care for Emily and Megan. But once the fifth week rolled around, Emily was alone, lonely, and starting to feel traces of the postpartum "baby blues." Nothing severe, but the sadness was enough to send her to a box of chocolates for consolation. She had read that a better diet could help, so fortunately she turned to NutriFit. I helped her structure her days so that she was eating her three meals and three snacks, planning exercise as an important part of her schedule, setting aside time for trips to the market, housework, cooking, and some gardening that she loves to do. Her days were full, her baby was thriving, and she even gave herself permission to take a little nap each day. Of the twenty-two pounds that were lingering five weeks after Megan's birth, twenty were gone in eight weeks. And she not only shed the weight, but eating right helped her lose the baby blues, too.

Since structure is one of the reasons working moms lose a little more quickly than mothers who stay home after childbirth, it's important for stay-at-home moms to keep to a schedule. Structure is a way for both you and your baby to thrive. A big part of Emily's success was that the *Body After Baby* plan showed her how to create structure in her life with three meals a day, two to three snacks, a short daily workout, a walk with baby, and a few mom-and-baby exercises. Baby's bath, naps, and nursing times can help add to the structure. When you commit to a schedule of healthy meals and appropriate healthy exercise, you'll see and feel the results quickly.

ALL MOMS DESERVE *BODY AFTER BABY*

Although many of my clients are movie stars, doctors, lawyers, and other top professionals, you don't have to have nannies, personal trainers, and chefs, or be rich *or* famous to achieve the nutrition and the activity levels these women attain. When my children were born, I, too, was a working woman who had to go back to work to help support my family. I honored my commitment to eating well and exercising daily. My children have grown up realizing how important it is to feed their bodies nutritiously. They're healthy, my husband's healthy, and I'm healthy.

My life was, and continues to be, extremely busy, multifaceted, and fulfilling. I achieved an appropriate postpartum weight and good muscle tone by following the same kind of sound nutritional regimen and exercise routine I've designed for my clients. Over the years I've fine-tuned the program to meet the needs of all types of working women and stay-at-home moms who need help. Now you can follow the plan at home, and fix easy recipes that will provide the nutrition your postpregnancy body craves.

The meal plans and recipes you'll find in these pages are the same that I use to feed hundreds of NutriFit clients every day. You'll also find important information from doctors and other health professionals whom I respect and admire. Plus, there are simple shopping lists to make your trips to the market efficient. You'll see that the healthful recipes I've included are simple to prepare, so you can devote less time to thinking about what to feed yourself and your family and more time to being with your baby. In the next two chapters, I'll give you a short course on Super

Fuel foods, the cornerstone of the *Body After Baby* plan, so you understand why you're eating what you're eating. Then I'll explain the specifics of the plan.

Whether you bought this book while pregnant or right after the baby was born, or you've been home with your baby for a few years, you're on your way to being lighter, healthier, and more fit, and you'll see results in thirty days. I know you're ready because you're reading this book. So let's get started now, and then, in one short month, you can get on the scale, look in your mirror, and check out your new *Body After Baby*!

the super fuel macronutrients: carbohydrates, proteins, fats, and water

MELINDA CAME TO ME when her son James was three months old. Her story wasn't new; it's just that she was the first new mom to tell me that she wanted a meal plan that was superhigh in protein, like the Atkins diet. She was so dedicated to her daily menu of fatty meat and cheese that I decided we had to have a long talk. Melinda was convinced that she would be able to lose her remaining twenty pounds of postpregnancy weight if she could only stick to this restrictive, almost no-carb approach. But she also admitted that right after James was born she had tried to eliminate carbs. She wasn't able to control her cravings for sweets, so she'd often splurge on candy and cookies—she just couldn't stick to a very low carbohydrate diet. She also noted that she often became weak on the high-protein diet and was frequently constipated.

I explained to Melinda that these were all typical symptoms of low-carb diets and that's why people don't have lasting success with them. I also explained how important a balanced food plan is for a new mother. I suggested that she try to incorporate some favorable grains along with some fruits and vegetables into her meals. She decided to give it a try. We started by adding hot, whole-grain cereal for breakfast, naturally sweetened by cooking it in half unsweetened juice and half water. Melinda began to look forward to eating fresh fruit in the evenings, finding that naturally sweet, juicy, fiber-filled apples, peaches, and oranges calmed her sweet tooth and allowed the cravings to pass. Her constipation disappeared almost immediately, since her increased fiber intake improved the functioning of her digestive tract. She was happier, healthier, and twenty pounds lighter in six weeks.

Jessica's idea of how to lose weight was just the opposite of Melinda's. She only ate carbohydrate-rich foods. At twenty-three years old and the mother of two young sons, she had gained nearly eighty pounds during her pregnancy. She lost about thirty-five pounds after the baby was born but was still struggling to lose the rest, plus was anemic and feeling very tired all the time. Jessica's biggest food issue was that she wasn't getting enough protein. She loved pasta, rice, potatoes, and bread—everything that she called "starchy and bad for you." She also couldn't stomach the thought of eating meat, the smell of fish, or the gamey taste she associated with poultry. We immediately started to work on her protein deficiency and anemia by adding vegetarian "meats" to her meals plus iron-rich leafy greens and legumes. At her doctor's suggestion, she also continued to supplement her diet with iron-rich prenatal vitamins. It wasn't long before Jessica was feeling stronger and more energetic. Her weight started to change, too, as she got control of her diet. It took a little longer than it usually does for most of our clients, but after about six months, Jessica was forty pounds lighter. And a year later, she was back to her prepregnancy weight. Most important, Jessica felt balanced and satisfied.

Both of these moms were in dietary trouble because they'd been sold on fad diets. Low-fat, high-fat, all-carb, low-carb, low-protein, all-protein, no-grain, whole-grain. For the last several years, we've all been bombarded with so many different fad diets that the terms carbohydrates, protein, and fat have taken on whole new meanings. Who wouldn't be confused? The fact is, and I have years of experience and can point to volumes of medical research to support my claim, the *only* eating plan that is healthy and truly effective for long-term weight loss, whether it's postpartum or not, is a plan that incorporates healthful levels of each. During the postpartum period, that balance is especially crucial.

That's what *Body After Baby* is all about: balance. You'll eat carbs, proteins, and fats in appropriate proportions, and you'll drink water throughout the day. Your body won't be craving nourishment because the foods you eat will supply it in a balanced, delicious way. You will find that when you eat a moderate diet that contains a combination of favorable carbs, proteins, fats, and water, you will have more mental focus and the weight will drop off at a healthy rate, plus you'll have more energy than you thought possible. That's because you'll be eating enough nutrient-dense calories in the Super Fuel foods I recommend. You won't run out of steam because you ate "empty" calories, the kind that are high in processed sugar and saturated fat. Super Fuel foods will keep you energized between meals. That's why Super Fuel foods are essential to the *Body After Baby* plan.

Carbohydrates

Let's start with a very simple explanation of the way the body uses carbohydrates: Carbohydrates are compounds of carbon, hydrogen, and oxygen that compose fiber, starches, and sugars. Fiber helps keep your digestive system working properly and aids the transport of nutrients through your body. Starches and sugars are the most effective nutrient source for energy because they're your body's primary source of glucose.

Glucose is the fuel for most of your body's cellular processes. It provides energy for your brain, your blood, your central nervous system, your eyes, and your kidneys. The body either uses glucose right away for energy or converts it to glycogen, which is then stored in the muscles for energy or converted to fat and stored in the liver. Once glucose is stored as fat, however, it can't be regenerated as glucose to feed the brain. This is one reason low-carbohydrate diets are dangerous. When there is a severe carb deficiency, your body has two problems: (1) The body has to turn to protein for energy, rather than letting the protein do its other vital jobs. (2) The body can't use its fats efficiently, since carbs are needed to combine with fat fragments to form energy. That's especially important for pregnant women to understand because when the body uses fat without the help of carbohydrates, it goes into a state of "ketosis," a condition in which unusual by-products, called ketones, accumulate in the blood. Ketosis during pregnancy can cause brain damage to the fetus and can cause irreversible mental retardation of the infant.

Yes, carbohydrates are an important part of everyone's daily menu to keep the body functioning properly. *But for a mother of a newborn, they couldn't be more important.*

Fiber and starches are called complex carbohydrates. These include leafy green vegetables, whole grains, and starchy vegetables such as potatoes, peas, and corn—and they're essential. Loaded with nutrition, they provide the necessary fuel to get through the day. They should not be avoided, no matter what any fad diet urges. A daily menu loaded with vegetables and whole grains will help you lose your pregnancy weight, heal your body, and keep your system working at its best. Fiber also plays a critical role in weight management; it contributes to feeling full, which allows you to eat less and still feel satisfied.

For you, right now, in the postpartum period, eating complex carbohydrates will help you lose weight because it allows insulin do its job. Insulin is the hormone that creates serotonin, the protein that helps you lose weight naturally if its levels are elevated after delivery. During the postpartum period, eating healthy complex carbohydrates increases insulin production, which in turn pushes the amino acid tryptophan from your blood into the brain, where it is used to help make serotonin. Only carbs can affect the hormones this way—not protein, not fat. And to keep your blood sugar constant and your serotonin level up the entire day, you want appropriate amounts of complex and healthy carbohydrates to build up serotonin.

Another hormone, leptin, is produced in the fat cells and sends messages to your brain that help curb your appetite and increase your metabolism. Leptin also plays an important part in the postpartum weight loss process. As UCLA endocrinologist Margaret England points out, "Eating complex carbohydrates helps to decrease your appetite through a complicated interrelationship between insulin and leptin. Exercise raises the leptin in your body thereby curbing the appetite, so if you eat more complex carbs such as vegetables, beans, and whole grains, exercise daily, and breast-feed for as long as you can, you will enhance the natural processes of losing weight postpartum."

There are other carbohydrates, known as simple carbohydrates, which don't have the same effect after a baby is born—or any time. Sweeteners (refined sugar, honey, corn syrup, etc.) and foods made with refined flours (even if they say "wheat" flour; they must say "whole wheat" to be considered a healthy choice), such as pasta, breads, cakes, and cookies, can be detrimental to your health, leading to diabetes, obesity, and, of course, tooth decay. These foods provide almost no nutritional value and help pack on pounds. They also have no effect on serotonin levels. Only complex carbohydrates affect serotonin levels.

Believe it or not, fat-free, low-calorie processed cookies and pastries that appear to be healthy often have more sugar than the regular versions to compensate for the lost flavor-enhancement properties of fat. Eating sugary foods can trigger a rush of insulin, which can cause blood sugar to drop dramatically. The result? Less energy, a bad mood, and almost instant hunger!

However, there are certainly some simple carbs that are healthy dietary choices.

Fruits, for example, have certain natural sugars, vitamins, minerals, and phyto-chemicals that are essential to good health. Likewise, milk and milk products are also simple carbohydrates that are important because they're infused with protein.

SUPER FUEL FRUITS AND VEGETABLES

I call fruits and vegetables "nature's botanical bounty." The body immediately benefits from the vitamins, minerals, fiber, and phytochemicals (all topics you'll read about in more detail in the next chapter) in these plant foods. They can also help fight off the ravages of many chronic diseases. Super Fuel fruits like apples can help lower the risk of heart disease, control diabetes, and prevent cancer and constipation. Berries are brimming with phytochemicals that may help prevent cataracts and cancer and reduce the risk of infection. Citrus fruits, kiwi, papayas, mangoes, and grapes are excellent sources of vitamin C and beta-carotene. Papayas also contain the enzyme papain, which can help ease upset stomach and ulcers. Toss some raisins into salads containing dark leafy greens for a vitamin C boost. They'll not only add potassium, iron, fiber, and folate, but they'll also allow the body to properly absorb the iron in the iron-rich greens. Your postpregnancy body is craving both fruits and vegetables because these Super Fuel foods help heal your body, protect it, and, of course, provide energy.

Vegetables virtually pump energy and disease-fighting nutrients into the body. Asparagus will help replenish the iron and folate you lost during pregnancy and birth. You can find a treasure trove of antioxidants in the colorful peppers, greens, and squashes; the antioxidants are thought to protect cells and promote healing throughout the body. Vegetables in the cruciferous family—such as broccoli, Brussels sprouts, bok choy, cabbage, cauliflower, Chinese cabbage, collard greens, horseradish, kale, kohlrabi, mustard greens, radish, rutabaga, turnips, and wasabi (not technically a vegetable, but made from the cruciferous vegetable horseradish)—help fight many diseases, including cancer, with high doses of fiber, phytonutrients, and minerals. These Super Fuel foods are particularly important when your body is recuperating after your baby is born. The leaves, or flowers, of these crispy vegetables have either four flowers (as in watercress), or grow from the base in the shape of a cross (like Brussels sprouts and broccoli), so they're easy to recognize at the market.

How do you choose the healthiest fruits and vegetables? Make choices from every spectrum of the rainbow. Generally speaking, the brighter their hue, the higher the vitamin and mineral content. And unlike foods from other parts of the food pyramid, more is better; studies show that as many as nine daily servings of vegetables and fruits is healthy on all fronts.

SUPER FUEL WHOLE GRAINS

Grains still account for most of the calories consumed by people worldwide. And that's a good thing, as long as you choose unrefined whole grains. Why do you want whole grains in their most natural state? The answer is simple. When grains are ground, milled, refined, and stripped of their constituent parts (such as bran, the fiber-rich outer layer; the germ, the part of the kernel with the most vitamins and protein; and the endosperm, which contains the most carbohydrates), nutrients are lost along the way. We're able to digest these refined grains more quickly, so hunger attacks sooner. Your body craves what whole grains can provide, especially postpartum. They're packed with complex carbohydrates, and provide the immediate energy necessary to fuel your muscles. When you replace highly refined carbohydrates with whole grains, you are receiving exactly what nature planned—delicious, nutritious, pure foods that are high in fiber. So always check for the words "whole grain" or "whole wheat," to be sure your grain is coming to you in the healthiest version possible.

Are these complex carbohydrates the enemy—bad for your health and waistline— as some fad diets would have you believe? Not a chance. Compared to an ordinary slice of white bread made with refined flour, a slice of whole-wheat bread, for instance, contains four times the amount of magnesium (which helps maintain the body's cells and enzymes), three times as much tissue-repairing zinc (which also plays a role in immune reactions, night vision, taste perception, and cell replication), and double the amount of potassium (an important blood-pressure regulator). Foods made with whole grains not only contain important vitamins and minerals, they also contain fiber and break down slowly when digested, which helps avoid damaging insulin spikes that negatively affect your mood. The carbs you should avoid overeating are found in white rice, white breads, and most types of commercially processed crackers, cookies, chips, soda, and candy bars. These carbohydrates (often referred to as "bad carbs") break down more quickly and can cause sugar overload.

The fiber in whole grains will help you to lose weight and will reduce your risk of obesity, heart disease, hypertension, and diabetes. These are important reasons to make whole grains an important part of your lifetime diet, not just your postpartum diet. Right now, some of the same aspects of fiber that help lower the risk of disease also help speed your healthy recovery from the birth of your child. Fiber binds cholesterol, which will help lower your cholesterol, and it slows the absorption of glucose into your bloodstream. This also aids in controlling your blood sugar levels and the resultant mood swings from high or low levels.

Keep complex carbohydrate portions appropriate (½ cup of whole-grain pasta or rice is considered a serving, as is one slice of bread), and aim for six servings per day. Combine these favorable carbs with fruits and vegetables, and you've got a winning combination for long-term health and weight management!

There are so many whole grains to choose from. The staples include brown rice, whole-wheat pasta, and cracked and steel-cut grains, such as oats, couscous, and bulgur. And there are alternative grains that are delicious and worth a try. Some of my favorites are amaranth, wild rice (a marsh grass), millet, and flaxseed. Flaxseed, which contains more lignans (antioxidants) than any other plant food, is most nutritious when the seeds are ground right before using. Sprinkle freshly ground seeds into muffin, bread, and cookie batters, and try a spoonful on top of your hot breakfast cereal. Flaxseed is also high in fiber and contains omega-3 fatty acids, which are additional cancer fighters.

In my menus I frequently include barley, which is easy to cook and versatile. It also has the lowest glycemic index value of all the grains, which means it is slowly digested and very gradually raises blood sugar—which helps delay hunger! Barley is healthy because of its tocotrienols (antioxidant members of the vitamin E family that help reduce damage to the body from free radicals), lignans (which help prevent blood clots), and soluble fiber. Buckwheat, bulgur, and their cousin, couscous, are whole-grain healers that help to lower cholesterol and decrease the risks of heart disease, cancer, and diabetes due to their high levels of fiber (bulgur and couscous) and flavonoids (buckwheat). Another whole grain, millet, contains magnesium that can help keep bones strong and ease premenstrual symptoms if you get them again. Millet also contains protein, helping to maintain your body's muscles, connective fibers, and other tissues.

But one grain that is almost unknown is one of the most delicious and nutritious: quinoa. Quinoa (pronounced "keen-wah") is rich in energy-boosting essential nutrients (iron, magnesium, and riboflavin) and has the highest level of protein of all of the grains. You'll find it in the whole grains section of almost any healthy-foods market. Rinse the quinoa under cold water until the water runs clear to remove the saponin, a naturally occurring coating on the grain that has a bitter flavor. It's simple to prepare; just add 1 cup of quinoa and a pinch of salt to 2 cups of boiling water. Cover the pan and let it simmer for twenty to thirty minutes (or until tender). Pour off any remaining water and it's ready to enjoy as you would any other grain.

Protein

Protein is the basis for every cell in our bodies. It's essential for growth, helping to build and repair skin, bones, muscles, organs, and blood and assisting in functions such as hormone production, immunity, blood clotting, and water balance. But like carbohydrates, fats, and water, it is only one of the important components of a healthy diet.

I don't want you to be misinformed the way Melinda was about the importance of protein. Tipping the balanced composition of your meals in favor of protein is counterproductive when you are trying to lose weight during the postpartum period. Your body is totally ready to lose weight; your hormones are working with you to drop pounds. Add too much protein to your diet and your hormones will be totally out of kilter. That's because in the first trimester postpartum, there is a critical interplay between the hormones serotonin and insulin and the amino acid tryptophan. If you introduce extreme amounts of protein, that interplay falls apart. Carbohydrates, not protein, cause the pancreas to produce insulin. Without carbohydrates, your insulin production decreases dramatically. And without insulin, tryptophan can't be channeled to the brain. The brain needs tryptophan to produce serotonin, which takes a big dip postpartum. Low levels result in postpartum depression, low energy, poor sleep, and guess what? Cravings for carbs. Your body will fight a high-protein diet during the postpartum period.

Don't be tempted to eat high-fat foods, either. Choosing more than 20–25 percent of your calories from fat, which has often been touted as the bonus on a high-protein diet, is a recipe for disaster. Excess fat in your daily food intake negatively affects your hormones and your mood, it encourages fatigue (*fat*-igue), and it has been proven time and again to promote weight gain.

However, eaten moderately, in combination with carbohydrates, fat, and water, protein increases your energy, helps lower your blood sugar, and encourages

healthy skin, nails, and hair. When you are breast-feeding, your body demands more protein than usual. While you need to consume only 46–50 grams of protein when you're not breast-feeding, you'll need at least 65 grams a day during lactation. Meat, poultry, and fish are great sources of complete proteins, meaning they include the nine essential amino acids (histidine, isoleucine, leucine, lysine, methionine, phenylalanine, threonine, tryptophan, and valine) that must be present for a complete protein to be formed. The plant proteins found in nuts, seeds, grains, legumes, and some fruits and vegetables are also wonderful nutritive sources, but they are not "complete" protein sources by themselves. When you eat whole grains with these favorable, higher protein foods derived from plants, you can create a complete protein (like those found in animal food sources). The whole grains and legumes don't necessarily need to be eaten at the same time; simply add them to your meal plan on the same day and your body will store and combine the amino acids to achieve the same benefits of complete animal proteins.

Protein from all sources should make up about 20–25 percent of your total daily calories. Be aware, though, that too much protein of any kind can leech calcium out of your body, and there is a concern that too much animal protein can lead to kidney and liver problems. Although it is possible that a high-protein diet might make it easier to slim down, it is generally a short-term solution if not accompanied by significant changes in long-term eating habits. So it's clearly not the best nutritional approach for postpartum moms.

Super Fuel Meat, Poultry, and Fish

Since postpartum women have lost a great deal of blood during delivery, iron-deficient anemia is not uncommon in new moms. Dietary iron is available in two forms: heme iron from meat, poultry, and fish and nonheme iron from plant sources. Our bodies absorb heme iron much more efficiently than nonheme iron. Lean red meat is a major source of heme iron, so it plays an important part in building healthy blood and muscle. Look for the leanest cuts of beef, those with "loin" in the name. Beef also contains riboflavin, or vitamin B_2, which supports normal skin and vision health, and helps release energy from the nutrients you eat. Another red meat, lamb, is a good source of zinc, which can promote faster wound healing and boost immunity from infections. Its heme iron level, which can help stave off anemia, is higher than that of chicken and other white meats. Because red meats are high in saturated fats, it makes sense to limit the amount you eat each week. Remember that red meat is an excellent protein source, so a little goes a long way.

Chicken is an important protein source for postpartum moms because of its abundance of niacin, a B vitamin that can help reduce cholesterol levels. Plus, its abundant level of B_6 helps make red blood cells and the "feel good" chemical serotonin. Turkey is also a good source of B_6, niacin, heme iron, and zinc. Pork, dubbed "the other white meat," is a lean protein source of thiamin (vitamin B_1) and has more heme iron than an equal serving of chicken.

Perhaps you've heard some controversy about eating fish. Seafood is not perfect, but the primary concern lies in the toxins that can concentrate in the flesh of oily fish. The heavy metal mercury is of particular concern. The larger fish, including swordfish, shark, tilefish, and king mackerel, have the highest levels of the toxin. Some can contain worrisome levels of PCBs (toxins called polychlorinated biphenyls). The amount of PCBs in fish depends on the waters where they were caught, so check with your fishmonger, or the head of the seafood department in your local market. Although not conclusive, present recommendations urge children and pregnant or nursing mothers to eat no more than 12 ounces of fish (two to three servings) a week and to completely avoid swordfish, shark, tilefish, and king mackerel. These large ocean fish consume smaller fish, which can lead to higher levels of contaminants.

Cold-water finfish (such as salmon, trout, tuna, whitefish, herring, and sardines) are protein sources that not only provide the benefits of protein, but they're also loaded with polyunsaturated fats known as omega-3 fatty acids, which are very heart-healthy. Shellfish, such as lobster, scallops, shrimp, and oysters, also contain omega-3s, which have been shown to dramatically reduce the risk of death from heart attack. These fish also contain vitamin B_{12} (which helps make red blood cells and keeps nerves healthy), zinc, iron, magnesium, and potassium. And don't forget that the little fish—herring and sardines—are high in omega-3s and low in toxins. I've included a number of omega-3-rich fish entrees in the *Body After Baby* meal plans to ensure that you'll get enough of these important fatty acids in your diet.

Our ancient ancestors hunted for their meat, poultry, and fish and expended a lot of energy doing so, using protein for building and maintaining muscle mass. With modern feedlots producing huge volumes of meats and poultry and grocery store meat counters offering convenient access, we don't have to be hunters anymore.

The result? We eat roughly twice as much protein as we need, risking injury to our kidneys and livers. Thus, it's important to consider portion size as well as frequency of consumption when including meat in your meals. The USDA considers 3 ounces of meat to be one serving of protein. That makes most restaurant portions large enough for several days' worth of protein. I recommend this weekly schedule for eating animal proteins: beef, veal, lamb, or pork once or twice a week; chicken or turkey twice a week; and fish and other seafood two to three times per week, plus up to four eggs a week.

SUPER FUEL EGGS, LEGUMES, NUTS, AND SOY

For moms of newborns, eggs provide another source of protein that has another important benefit—they're quick and easy to prepare. Plus, eggs are loaded with vitamins A and B_{12}, folic acid, and riboflavin. One of the best bargains in the grocery store is a carton of those "incredible, edible" eggs. According to the USDA, Americans consumed 374 eggs per capita in 1959, and 250 in 2000, an indication that consumers are conscious of the cholesterol levels in egg yolks. But that doesn't mean you should give up this important protein source. Quite the contrary. Although an egg yolk contains twice the cholesterol of a 3-ounce serving of beef, three or four eggs can be safely consumed each week in a healthy diet. You can also safely use egg substitutes, which are made from egg whites and are generally fat- and cholesterol-free.

Legumes are seeds harvested from pod-bearing plants—think soybeans, peas, and green beans—and they're a powerhouse of protein. They also contain energy-boosting carbohydrates and fiber, are low in fat, and are packed with minerals. Other important legumes are kidney, black, white, red, pinto, and garbanzo beans. Regardless of which you choose, you can't beat beans for filling up the healthy way, reducing your risk of overeating and thus aiding greatly in weight control. Here's a cooking tip that will benefit everyone, but especially postpartum moms: soaking beans before you cook them removes most of the beans' gas-producing sugars (called oligosaccharides). First sort the beans to remove any foreign matter. Rinse thoroughly and soak the beans in cold water overnight. Drain the water and put the beans in a pot of fresh water to cover by about three inches. Add a bit of salt and bring the water to a slow boil. Cook the beans until soft, then drain in a colander. Spread the beans on a cookie sheet to cool.

Lentils are frequently used as a meat substitute in main dishes. Unlike beans, lentils don't require soaking before cooking, a big plus to cooks who are in a hurry. In addition to protein, lentils contain iron and folate, as well as vitamins A and B, phosphorus, and bone-friendly calcium. This high-fiber food helps alleviate constipation naturally. Any water that's left after you cook the lentils will be rich in B vitamins, so use it when your recipes call for liquid, or save it for your next soup.

Nuts make great snacks for postpartum moms, as they can be eaten "on the go." Peanuts, a perennial favorite, aren't actually nuts at all, but legumes. They're rich in protein, providing a vegetarian energy source. So, if you're looking for a satisfying meal that's a complete protein, you should try all-natural peanut butter (the reduced-fat variety is worth seeking out) on whole wheat bread. Peanuts also contain the monounsaturated and polyunsaturated healthy fats that help reduce the risk of heart disease and cancer.

Soy is an increasingly popular source of protein. While scientists continue to research the health benefits of soy with respect to disease risk reduction, they have already determined that soy foods are the richest dietary source of phytochemicals that may help lower cholesterol. In fact, if a soy product contains 6.25 grams of soy protein per serving and is eaten as part of a low-fat diet that includes 25 grams of soy protein a day, FDA-approved labeling says the product can lower the cholesterol levels of people suffering from high cholesterol. The diverse and powerful phytochemicals in soy foods may also help reduce the risk of certain breast and colon cancers, heart disease, and osteoporosis. Aside from soybeans (also known as edamame), which can be found frozen, fresh, canned, dried, and roasted, you can drink, cook, and bake with soy milk (made from ground, soaked soybeans) in place of cow's milk. Tempeh, which is made from fermented soybean cakes, and tofu, made from coagulated soybean curd, are available in several forms and can be used in a variety of ways in cooking and baking and in their natural state.

SUPER FUEL LOW-FAT DAIRY

The *Body After Baby* menus contain abundant amounts of dairy, helping to replenish the calcium your body used to form your baby's bones. Dairy products play an important role in a healthy diet. Milk and its counterparts (yogurt, cheese, cottage cheese, and even ice cream) are good sources of protein. One cup of fat-free milk, for instance, has more protein than a large egg or an ounce of ham. Calcium-rich dairy is critical for building bones and helping to lower cholesterol and blood pressure levels, but always reach for low-fat or fat-free products—they contain the same beneficial nutrients without the artery-clogging saturated fat. Generally, the harder the cheese, the lower the fat, so keep Parmesan and Romano close at hand. Yogurt that contains live and active cultures can help strengthen the immune system and help keep your digestive tract healthy. Go for plain yogurt and add your own fresh fruit for the healthiest version.

Fat

For more than forty years, most researchers have agreed that the optimal diets were those that were low in fat. Today, research shows that certain types of fat, found in foods like fish, olive oil, avocados, and walnuts, actually improve levels of good cholesterol (HDL) and significantly reduce the risk of heart disease. Fat is an essential part of anyone's diet, and new research shows that it can even aid in weight loss. Healthy fats, such as those found in olive oil, avocados, walnuts, and almonds, provide energy, insulate against extreme temperatures, protect our organs, and keep our skin healthy. These "good" fats also seem to delay hunger pangs. But even good fats contain more than double the calories (containing 9 calories per gram) of either proteins or carbohydrates (containing 4 calories per gram). There are many theories about what the optimal amount of fat in a healthy diet should be, but even if you allow for 20–30 percent of your daily calories from favorable fat sources, there's little room for error. Too much fat, even favorable fat, sends your calorie intake zooming out of control. You'll find sufficient amounts of fat in the *Body After Baby* plan to keep your body working efficiently and to keep your hunger at bay.

Monounsaturated and polyunsaturated fats are good for you. They not only help lower your risk of heart disease, but they may reduce breast cancer risk. Both of these fats, found in vegetable (think olive, safflower, and canola) and nut/seed oils (I especially like peanut, sesame, and sunflower oils), are rich in vitamin E, which can stop the cellular damage that can lead to cancer.

Omega-3—a polyunsaturated fatty acid found in some fish, walnuts, soybeans, and flaxseed—has been shown to reduce clotting and inflammation in arteries, which can help lower heart disease and stroke risk. Let's distinguish omega-3 fatty acids from omega-6 fatty acids, which come from sources such as nuts, seeds, whole grains, margarine, and certain vegetable oils, including corn, soybean, and safflower oils. Because you are exposed to so many of these polyunsaturated fatty acids in your daily diet (estimates are that most people in the United States eat nine times as many omega-6 fatty acids), it's wise to limit your intake of omega-6 fatty acids.

As for "bad" fats, the saturated fats found in meats, lard, and full-fat dairy products are notorious for raising levels of artery-clogging LDL cholesterol. These naturally occurring unfavorable fats should be eaten only in small amounts. Too much saturated fat will increase your risk of obesity, diabetes, cancer, gall bladder disease, and arthritis. Eating too much saturated fat also sets a poor dietary pattern for your new baby and your entire family. Once you acquire a "fat tooth," it can be as bad for your body as a "sweet tooth"—or worse.

You should also avoid all trans fat, which is made from partially hydrogenated fats and oils. Trans fats can clog arteries and raise cholesterol—especially the LDL cholesterol—just like saturated fats. Trans fat is found in vegetable shortening, stick margarine, crackers, cookies, snack foods, and other foods made with or fried in partially hydrogenated oils. So rely on the healthier canola and olive oils for cooking and salad dressing.

BREAST-FEEDING AND FAT

Infants need fat in their diets, and they get it in sufficient quantities from breast milk. More than half the calories of breast milk come from fat. The composition of breast milk composition changes constantly, based on your diet and your environment. The fat content of your breast milk can change throughout the course of a day. The earliest form of milk you provide for the baby, colostrum, contains proportionally greater amounts of protein and minerals and less fat than mature milk. As your infant ages, the fat content of the milk increases. So it makes sense that the fat in your body becomes essential when you are breast-feeding. Although producing milk uses the fat in your daily diet first, it will also rely on the fat stored in your body. So if you limit the fat you ingest to a healthy 20–25 percent of your daily caloric intake, your fat stores will quickly be put into action. Sometimes even the fat that accumulated in your body prior to your pregnancy will be used to provide the appropriate nutrition for the baby. Studies have demonstrated that breast-feeding mothers tend to lose more weight when their babies are three to six months old than formula-feeding mothers who are actually consuming fewer calories. That's probably because the breast-feeding moms are producing more milk to nourish their growing babies, so their own fat stores are being depleted.

Water

Water completes our discussion of essential nutrients. Indeed, your body can't function without it. Present in every cell of the body, water constitutes 60–75 percent of your body weight, about 10 to 12 gallons. Drinking water is especially important after the baby is born because it carries nutrients to the cells and removes toxins and waste products. Moreover, it helps your body get back to total health by helping to stabilize body temperature and maintain its blood volume. Every day the average person loses about 3.5 percent of her body weight (or about 2½ quarts of water) in urine, perspiration, and other body fluids, but when you are lactating you lose even more. I recommend that you drink one to three glasses of water per hour. Even if you don't feel thirsty, it's especially important to drink water since it takes a long time for your brain to get the message from your body that its water stores are depleted. Most women are thirsty when they're breast-feeding because the body is using more water than it's taking in. So make a healthy pledge to yourself, and drink a minimum of one cup of water every waking hour and you'll keep yourself well hydrated. This will also ensure that your breast milk will continue to flow properly. If you do get thirsty, respond with water, not the empty calories of sodas. Sodas of all kinds, whether naturally sweetened or artificially sweetened, contain chemicals that may not be good for you, so it's best to avoid them completely, if possible.

The Bottom Line

Here's a summary of the top six nutrition points I'd like you to remember and incorporate into your daily menu planning:

1. A balance of favorable fats, complex carbohydrates, and protein is the key to short- and long-term weight management.
2. Whole grains provide critical fiber and energy to keep your body functioning properly.
3. Vegetables and fruits are nutrient-rich complex carbohydrates that are abundant in fiber and water.
4. Fish contains the healthy omega-3 fats your body needs. "Go fishing" for dinner

two to three times a week, but avoid shark, swordfish, tilefish, and king mackerel because of their high mercury content.

5. There are healthy fats and there are unhealthy fats. Opt for monounsaturated and polyunsaturated fats and avoid saturated fats and trans fats whenever possible.

6. When you're nursing you need to drink water frequently. Drink at least one cup an hour, more if you can. Remember, your body needs water before your brain registers thirst. When you're not breast-feeding, drink water and eat foods that contain a high percentage of water to keep your body properly hydrated. Water keeps your satiation level high and your calorie intake low.

nature's pharmacy:
super fuel micronutrients

MARCY HAD A particularly difficult time during her pregnancy because she was suffering from multiple sclerosis. For nine months her energy was zapped. When she started at NutriFit, she had just given birth to a healthy, happy baby boy. But Marcy was exhausted and worried that she wouldn't have enough energy to care for her child. I planned her meals carefully, making sure that everything she ate was optimal fuel for her body. From Day 1 she ate three meals a day and three snacks. She noticed a difference immediately. "Eating regularly, six times a day, definitely impacts my energy levels," Marcy explains. On weekends, she found that she would get off her regular schedule and she'd feel it right away: "When I don't eat as often, I find myself scrounging around in the fridge and I notice I don't feel as well. Having the food right in front of me makes a big difference not only in my energy levels but also in my overall sense of well-being."

Marcy didn't realize it at first, but her energy was depleted because she wasn't eating the right foods. Couple that with MS and it's amazing that she was able to move around at all during her pregnancy. The key to high energy for every mom is right in nature's pharmacy of Super Fuel foods. With a little knowledge, you can select foods rich in nutrients that enhance your health, and when you choose those Super Fuel foods you are getting critical macronutrients, the four essential nutrients that nourish your body—water, proteins, carbohydrates, and fats. But perhaps even more important, you ensure that you're getting your essential micronutrients, the vitamins and minerals that help meet your body's needs during the postpartum period. Yes, you'll take the multivitamin your doctor recommends, of course. But many of the essential phytochemicals (biologically active substances found in plants) are not adequately contained in supplements or cannot be absorbed properly by the body in pill form. The more micronutrients you get from whole food sources, the healthier your body will be.

Think of this chapter as a short course in postpregnancy nutrition that will help you select foods that give you the most bang for the bite, foods that are exceptionally rich in those all-important micronutrients. You've already been exposed to plenty of information about the sources of vitamins and minerals. For instance, you know that milk has vitamin D, citrus fruits are excellent sources of vitamin C, and spinach provides iron (Popeye was right!). But did you know that citrus also contains beta-carotene, a powerful antioxidant, and so does spinach, which is also

can you get all your vitamins and minerals from food?

AFTER DELIVERY, the nursing mom needs about 500 extra calories a day for lactation. But packing all the nutrition you need in those 500 calories takes careful planning, leaving little extra room for goodies. The idea is to consume foods with the most nutrients for the fewest calories. This means cutting excess fats and sweets, so your calories are coming from food sources with the most vitamins, minerals, and phytonutrients. For example, a quart of nonfat milk will provide your daily calcium needs for about 350 calories, but if you drink whole milk, it will set you back 600 calories! Similarly, 6 ounces of chicken breast has 300 calories and helps to meet your protein needs, but 6 ounces of steak has twice the calories. Choose low-calorie, nutrient-dense whole fruits, steamed vegetables, and whole grains. Two servings of fortified whole-grain cereals can help to meet iron needs, which are so important after delivery.

You should discuss with your doctor the need to continue your prenatal vitamins after delivery. Most women like to combine food sources with the "insurance" of the vitamins to make sure they are meeting needs. There is no risk of consuming too many vitamins or minerals from foods, but supplements should be taken according to directions to avoid taking too much. Postpartum moms who choose not to nurse have lower calorie requirements, and still need nutrient-dense, low-calorie foods to help keep energy levels up and to assist with post-baby weight loss.

—SUSAN BOWERMAN, M.S., R.D.
Assistant Director, UCLA Center for Human Nutrition
University of California—Los Angeles

a great source of calcium? Or that rice and potatoes will help you sleep better while your body's healing? By the time you're done reading this chapter, you'll know which foods are a good, natural source of vitamin E and which ones will provide essential vitamins and minerals like B$_{12}$ and folic acid. And, most important, after forty anticipation-filled weeks of wear and tear on your body, you'll know how to eat your way to strength.

I call them "marvelous micronutrients" because these vitamins and minerals do so much to heal our bodies. As you read on, you'll see which foods will give you the healthy body you want as a new mom.

Value Your Vitamins

Marie Osmond, who is the mother of eight children, used NutriFit to provide meals when filming her daytime talk show with her brother Donny. While both of them had healthy eating habits, Marie's needs were a little more challenging since she was avoiding both wheat and dairy products, two sources of important vitamins and minerals. We put Marie on the *Body After Baby* plan to help ensure her intake of vitamin D and calcium. While the plan features generous quantities of calcium-rich dairy, we fortified her menus with dark leafy greens and soy products. The results? A beautiful star, a healthy body, and a happy mom.

Our bodies just don't produce all of the vitamins that are necessary for optimal health. We need to get them elsewhere or our systems simply can't function properly. That's especially true right after baby is born. After delivery your body's store of vitamins is depleted and the energy you expend now while caring for baby is a continual drain. The best sources of replenishment for these important micronutrients are the foods you eat. Multivitamin supplements cover the basics, so don't forget to take yours daily, but every expert I've ever spoken to agrees that there's no pill that really substitutes for the bounty of vitamins you get from well-chosen food. What nature puts together is a package of vitamins and minerals that's also rich in fiber and water and calories, all of which add up to Super Fuel for the body. As a new mom, your body needs the whole package to operate efficiently.

We've talked about the huge changes your body has gone through during pregnancy. Micronutrients make a huge difference, not just in the healing process, but in restoring your strength. Pregnancy can wreak havoc with your bones, since so many of the nutrients that build bones go directly to the growing baby. That's one of the important reasons your health-care provider insists on a good multivitamin during your pregnancy. After the baby is born you'll want to continue "feeding" your bones to avoid osteoporosis in the future.

Many people think that adding more calcium to your diet is enough. But there are important vitamin interactions in the bone development process. Vitamin B_{12}, for instance, is not just helpful for increasing your energy; it also helps build stronger bones. A recent Tufts University study of more than 2,500 men and women showed that low levels of vitamin B_{12} correlated with low bone density. Likewise, vitamin K activates a protein that helps calcium crystallize, which, in turn, strengthens the matrix of the bone. Your careful attention to the amount of calcium you get now *and* the vitamins and minerals that support it in your body will start your fight against future osteoporosis.

Vitamin D is essential to properly absorbing and using calcium and phosphorus, another key aspect of protecting your bones. If you're nursing, vitamin D is going to be of utmost importance to your baby's development. Vitamin D can be detrimental to the body if you consume too much, so the best source is not a supplement. Since our bodies produce vitamin D when we are exposed to sunlight, the sun and the food we eat are the best sources of this essential nutrient. After all those warnings about too much sun exposure, medical researchers now urge us to spend five to ten minutes in the sun every day *without* sunscreen, so our bodies can naturally absorb vitamin D from the rays. (That's not license to burn; too much unprotected exposure to the sun's ultraviolet light will definitely damage your skin and can result in skin cancers.) You can also get your vitamin D by drinking fortified milk or orange juice, or by eating eggs, canned tuna, or fortified cereals.

Vitamin A helps cells mature, which means that as you are healing and your body is returning to its prepregnancy state, foods high in beta-carotene (which the body converts to vitamin A), such as apricots, asparagus, broccoli, spinach, and other green and yellow fruits and vegetables, will provide enough vitamin A to help mend tissues and provide immunity against debilitating colds and flu. Although vitamin A is essential for bone growth—both yours and your baby's—too much can be destructive to bones and may actually contribute to the development of osteoporosis. Like vitamins E, D, and K, vitamin A is fat-soluble and tends to be stored in the body's fatty tissue. Too much A can be toxic to your liver. That's why it's so beneficial to eat foods that are high in beta-carotene rather than taking pills; you can't overdose, but you still get its health benefits.

Did you know that a deficiency of vitamin C can lead to severe fatigue? That's the last thing you need now, so it makes sense to eat plenty of the fruits and vegetables that are packed with C. Munch those red and yellow bell peppers, snack on berries, and eat at least one citrus fruit daily! Because vitamin C and the B vitamins are water-soluble they are eliminated regularly by your body, so they need constant replenishment. In addition to being a fatigue fighter, the antioxidant vitamin C is necessary for tissue growth and its repair. It causes the body to form collagen, the most prevalent protein in the body, responsible for strong blood vessels and skin (yes, it is a stretch-mark and wrinkle fighter!). While vitamin C isn't getting all the publicity that it once did, its list of health benefits goes on and on, from fighting virus infections like the common cold to helping to reduce high blood pressure. Foods that are packed with C are a postpregnancy must.

The Bs are eight vitamins that work together to keep your metabolism at its peak. A combination of vitamin B_9 (commonly called folate or folic acid), plus vitamins B_6 and B_{12}, helps lower homocysteine levels in the body, which in turn benefits memory and visual perception, both of which can play tricks on you when you're stressed by a new routine. Fortunately the Bs are naturally available in all sorts of foods. Because they can be destroyed when foods are cooked, it's important to eat plenty of raw vegetables and fruits that contain them (see chart that follows).

Your body will need more vitamin Є after the baby is born if you are breast-feeding, especially the first few days. That's because colostrum, the rich yellow milk your baby will drink from your breast during early lactation, is not only rich in protein and immune factors, but also vitamin Є. So even though the body can store the fat-soluble vitamin, breast-feeding can deplete the stores. Rather than taking supplements, increase your intake of foods that are rich in Є, such as nuts and dark leafy green vegetables. I make that recommendation because taking vitamin Є supplements has been the subject of great debate in the medical community, since one recent study showed the supplements are perfectly safe and another suggested that taking 400 units per day may be linked to premature death. Both studies are subject to interpretation, but it's safest to fulfill your vitamin needs by eating wholesome, natural foods rich in micronutrients. In fact, in 2004 the American

Heart Association began discouraging the use of supplements of any antioxidant vitamin—E, C, or beta-carotene—in favor of eating a healthy diet rich in the natural vitamins. It's a moderate approach, with great benefits.

Here's a chart that shows the most recent data on major vitamins, why you need them when you're postpartum, and the most common food sources for each.

VITAMIN	WHY YOU NEED IT NOW MORE THAN EVER	FOOD SOURCE
A	Increases bone strength; increases resistance to viral infection; boosts the immune system; repairs epithelial tissues that cover the whole surface of the body	Liver, fish liver oils, fortified milk, eggs, sweet potatoes, pumpkin, carrots, lentils, dark green leafy vegetables
B₁ (thiamine)	Increases energy; keeps cells and nerves healthy	Oysters, green peas, brewer's yeast, lean pork, dried beans and peas, collard greens, oranges, wheat germ, breads and cereals, whole grains, peanuts and peanut butter
B₂ (riboflavin)	Increases energy; helps maintain strength of bones; is essential to production and regulation of hormones and formation of red blood cells	Dairy, meat, poultry, fish, enriched and fortified grains, cereals and bakery products, green vegetables such as broccoli, turnip greens, asparagus, and spinach
B₃ (niacin)	Increases energy; aids breakdown of protein and fats; helps synthesize fats and certain hormones; aids formation of red blood cells	Meat, poultry, fish, enriched cereals and grains, nuts. Milk and eggs contain very little niacin but they provide tryptophan, which is converted into niacin by the body.
B₅ (pantothenic acid)	Fights stress by helping the body produce adrenal hormones as well as antibodies; increases stamina; aids digestive system	Beef, nuts, vegetables, eggs, legumes, whole-wheat and rye flour, brewer's yeast, saltwater fish
B₆ (pyridoxine)	Accelerates formation of red blood cells; allows breakdown of carbohydrates, fats, and proteins; helps process amino acids and maintain nervous system; helps reduce water retention; regulates hormones	Chicken, fish, kidney, liver, pork, eggs, brown rice, soybeans, oats, whole-wheat products, peanuts, walnuts
Folate (also called folacin) and its component folic acid (an essential B vitamin)	Prevents anemia by producing and maintaining cells and the cells' genetic codes (RNA and DNA); aids formation of red and white blood cells in the bone marrow; fights fatigue	Red meat, salmon or tuna, chicken, barley, bran and other whole grains, brewer's yeast, brown rice, dairy products, dark green leafy vegetables and root vegetables, legumes, liver, yeast

VITAMIN	WHY YOU NEED IT NOW MORE THAN EVER	FOOD SOURCE
B₁₂ (cyanocobalamin)	Aids in production of red blood cells and in metabolism of carbohydrates, protein, and fat for the normal production of amino acids; helps maintain nervous system; regulates hormones	Brewer's yeast, clams, eggs, seafood, milk and dairy products, soy products, alfalfa
C (ascorbic acid)	Fights stress; helps produce collagen; contributes to maintenance of capillaries, bones, and teeth	Green and red peppers, collard greens, broccoli, spinach, tomatoes, potatoes, strawberries, oranges and other citrus, papaya, kiwi, grapes, berries
D	Regulates the absorption and use of calcium and phosphorus; maintains healthy nerve and muscle systems	Sunlight, fortified milk, trans fat–free margarine, eggs, butter
E	Protects fats and vitamin A in the body from destruction; stabilizes cell membranes; protects tissues	Nuts and seeds, green leafy vegetables, wheat germ, cold-pressed vegetable oils, sweet potatoes, brown rice, cornmeal, eggs, kelp, milk, organ meats, whole grains
K	Regulates blood clotting; aids bone formation and healing; helps metabolize glucose	Asparagus, blackstrap molasses, cruciferous vegetables (broccoli, Brussels sprouts, cabbage, cauliflower), dark green leafy vegetables, egg yolks, liver, liver, oats, rye, safflower oil, soybeans, wheat
Biotin	Breaks down fats, amino acids, and carbohydrates; contributes to cell growth; relieves muscle pain	Liver, egg yolk, soy flour, whole grains, brewer's yeast
Choline	Aids in brain and nerve function, hormone production, and liver function; facilitates metabolism of fat and cholesterol	Egg yolks, lecithin, legumes, meat, dairy, soy, whole grains

FREE RADICALS AND ANTIOXIDANTS

You've undoubtedly heard the term "antioxidant." It refers to vitamins that protect cells from damage caused by free radicals (another much-used term) that are produced in our bodies and in the environment by pollutants such as car exhaust and smoke from cigarettes and industrial facilities. During the postpartum period arming yourself with antioxidants will fortify your immune system when you need it the most—now!

Free radicals are a by-product of a destructive oxidation process that goes on in our bodies. Think of it like the oxidation that causes rust on metal or makes food go bad. If our bodies create too many free radicals, the cellular damage can result in problems like cancer and heart disease. Right after your baby is born, you're more vulnerable to stress, and antioxidants are powerful stress fighters. The emotional stress of dealing with your newly expanded family can increase the amount of free radicals in your body, so it's important to eat antioxidant-rich foods to combat that stress.

Many researchers believe that antioxidant vitamins such as A, C, E, and beta-carotene, and the minerals selenium, zinc, manganese, copper, and iron may help reduce blood pressure, raise levels of good cholesterol (HDL), and reduce the levels of bad cholesterol. That's a huge plus postpregnancy, since during pregnancy many women see their blood pressure and cholesterol levels zoom upward. Here's where eating your nutrients, instead of the hassle of combining numerous supplements, makes a big difference. Why take a handful of pills when you can get your antioxidants from food? A single multivitamin and a minimum of five servings of fruits and veggies (but preferably seven to nine) will assure you of maintaining appropriate levels of disease-fighting antioxidants. The other bonus is that filling up on these nutritious but low-calorie foods will mean that your fiber intake is high, and your satisfaction level is even higher. When I'm planning meals, I include several foods that contain antioxidants—they're Super Fuel foods that I believe in. Here's my list:

The Top Antioxidant Fruits and Vegetables

Berries (blackberries, blueberries, raspberries, strawberries)	Mango	Cherries	Broccoli
	Prunes	Sweet potatoes	Garlic
	Raisins	Yams	Red bell pepper
Papaya	Plums	Kale	Onion
Cantaloupe	Oranges	Spinach	Corn
Watermelon	Red grapes	Brussels sprouts	Eggplant

Maximize Your Minerals

Minerals are key to your body's optimal performance and they are essential to your baby's health. So if you are nursing, you must be doubly conscious of your mineral intake to be certain your breast milk is supernutritious. The *Body After Baby* plan is a mineral-rich diet that draws on the nutrients that occur naturally in dairy products, poultry, meat, fish, whole grains, fruits, and vegetables. Taking mineral supplements can be confusing, so be certain if you want to pursue taking supplements that you rely on guidance from a specialist. But first, see how you feel after just a week on *Body After Baby,* where your minerals come right from the food in the meal plan!

When Chris came to NutriFit, she was four months postpartum, breast-feeding, and suffering from terrible fatigue. Her doctor told her that she had severe anemia and a compromised immune system caused by iron deficiency. Chris had a weight problem too: she was losing too much weight too fast, and getting weaker by the day. She wasn't sure that she could continue breast-feeding or caring for her baby because she was too tired all the time. The fatigue was overwhelming. With her doctor's approval, I acted quickly and put Chris on the *Body After Baby* plan, adding extra calories to suit her unique needs. In less than thirty days Chris was experiencing noticeable improvement in her energy levels. Balancing Chris's minerals took longer than with some clients, but in about two months her condition stabilized and she was on the mend. Because she was getting the proper nutrition, from Day 1 on the plan, she was able to continue successfully breast-feeding and taking care of her little one. With the proper nutritional guidance, Chris learned about her specific dietary needs and changed her eating habits completely. Once she was able to manage her mineral intake with wholesome foods, she knew she could push through anything.

Bulk Minerals and Trace Minerals

Minerals are divided into two groups. One group, bulk minerals, includes minerals most moms have heard of: calcium, magnesium, sodium, potassium, and phosphorus. Your body needs relatively large amounts of these bulk minerals to get their full benefits. The others are called trace minerals and you need minute amounts to accomplish major things in your body. You may be aware of many of these, such as iron, iodine, and zinc; but the function of many others, such as boron, chromium, copper, germanium, manganese, molybdenum, selenium, silicon, sulfur, and vanadium, may be less familiar.

Since when you are nursing you are constantly diverting the calcium from your body to help build your baby's bones, you must consume enough calcium to meet your body's needs, too. You'll see the results of the calcium baby gets each day as he or she gets longer and stronger and grows teeth (you nursing moms will notice those new little teeth right away—ouch!). So every bit of milk, yogurt, and dark leafy greens that you consume will be put to use.

I've talked about the weight loss that naturally occurs the day baby is born. In addition to the other weight loss, women lose about three pounds of blood. That's a huge loss of iron in your body—and it explains the fatigue you're probably feeling. When iron is depleted, you feel drained immediately—a very common problem for new moms. Restoring that iron will make you feel more energetic, since it helps to replenish the red blood cells. It also helps improve your concentration. Iron promotes collagen production, which is integral to the structure of the bone. The food you eat will help normalize your iron levels; besides the well-known sources such as lean red meat, fish, and poultry, you'll also get iron from delicious treats like beans, whole-grain cereal, dried apricots, and raisins.

The chart on the following page shows the important functions of bulk and trace minerals in your postpregnancy diet. You can select the foods listed to increase these minerals in your daily meals.

WHAT YOUR LACTATING BODY NEEDS

If you are breast-feeding you have specific dietary needs that you must meet and understand. Breast milk provides for your child's nutrition first—that's nature's way. Just as a mother's body provides whatever the baby needs during pregnancy, your body will produce enough nutritious breast milk to allow your baby to flourish. But just as in pregnancy, your energy levels and mood can suffer in this process of constant giving. But the nutrition of the *Body After Baby* plan can help.

The calories your body uses to produce 23 ounces of milk for your baby each day will add up to a natural weight loss of more than one pound per week. That's a simple equation of calories taken in and calories expended. However, you've got to be certain that the calories you eat are all nutrient-rich. The chart on page 41 is a breakdown of the nutrients you need each day while breast-feeding.

| --- | --- | --- |
Bulk Minerals		
Calcium	Increases and maintains bone mass; keeps teeth strong; aids blood clotting	Dairy products, tofu, seeds, dark green leafy vegetables
Magnesium	Assists in absorption of calcium and potassium; helps prevent depression; helps the body to relax; alleviates muscle weakness	Milk, apples, apricots, avocados, bananas, blackstrap molasses, cantaloupe, garlic, grapefruit, dark green leafy vegetables, sesame seeds, nuts, peaches, wheat germ, whole grains
Sodium	Helps to regulate the water and pH balance in the body; too much can cause high blood pressure, edema, and liver and kidney disease. An imbalance of sodium and potassium can lead to heart disease.	All foods contain some sodium
Phosphorous	Aids bone and tooth formation; enhances cell growth; helps strengthen contractions of heart muscle; helps body get energy from the food it takes in	Carbonated beverages, asparagus, fish, red meats, poultry, dairy products, eggs, whole grains, nuts, seeds
Potassium	Helps regulate blood pressure, important during breast-feeding period since your blood pressure may be elevated and doctors discourage nursing mothers from taking blood pressure medication	Bananas, apricots, avocados, blackstrap molasses, brewer's yeast, dairy products, fish, meat, potatoes, poultry, raisins, winter squash, soy products, tomatoes, wheat bran and other whole grains
Trace Minerals		
Chromium	Helps metabolize sugar for energy; aids synthesis of cholesterol, fats, and protein for energy; stabilizes blood sugar levels; prevents depression, fatigue, and glucose intolerance	Whole grains, wheat germ, cheese, brown rice, meat
Copper	Maintains the integrity of tissue; aids in formation of bones and red blood cells	Almonds, avocados, barley
Iodine	Helps formation of thyroid hormones, which regulate metabolism	Seafood and iodized salt
Iron	Protects body against anemia; helps formation of red blood cells; helps carry oxygen to muscles	Meat, raisins, dried apricots, potato skins, dried peas and beans
Manganese	Aids bone growth, protein and fat metabolism; stabilizes blood sugar; helps form cartilage and synovial fluid of the joints	Nuts and seeds, dark green leafy vegetables, avocados, blueberries, dried peas, pineapples, egg yolks

The *Body After Baby* plan is carefully formulated to match these nutrient goals so that you and your baby are properly nourished. This chart indicates that a nursing mom's nutrient needs change after the first six months of lactation. It reflects an assumption that your baby will begin getting food from sources other than breast milk and thus not drinking as much milk, so your body won't be making as much. If you're not supplementing your child's diet with solid food or commercial formula after six months, your nutrient requirements will remain the same until you decide to add supplemental nutrition to the baby's diet. Dark green leafy veggies, whole grains, and protein sources (especially fish) help you meet your need for these often overlooked but highly important nutrients.

NUTRIENT	WOMEN 25–50	PREGNANT WOMEN	LACTATING (0–6 MONTHS)	LACTATING (6–12 MONTHS)
Protein	50 g	60 g	65 g	62 g
Vitamin A	800 mcg RE	800 mcg RE	1,300 mcg RE	1,200 mcg RE
Vitamin D	5 mcg	10 mcg	10 mcg	10 mcg
Vitamin E	8 mg	10 mg	12 mg	11 mg
Vitamin K	65 mcg	65 mcg	65 mcg	65 mcg
Vitamin C	60 mg	70 mg	95 mg	90 mg
Thiamin	1.1 mg	1.5 mg	1.6 mg	1.6 mg
Riboflavin	1.3 mg	1.6 mg	1.8 mg	1.7 mg
Niacin	15 mg	17 mg	20 mg	20 mg
Vitamin B_6	1.6 mg	2.2 mg	2.1 mg	2.1 mg
Folic acid	180 mcg	400 mcg	280 mcg	260 mcg
Vitamin B_{12}	2.0 mcg	2.2 mcg	2.6 mcg	2.6 mcg
Calcium	800 mg	1,200 mg	1,200 mg	1,200 mg
Phosphorus	800 mg	1,200 mg	1,200 mg	1,200 mg
Magnesium	280 mg	320 mg	355 mg	340 mg
Iron	15 mg	30 mg	15 mg	15 mg
Zinc	12 mg	15 mg	19 mg	16 mg
Iodine	150 mcg	175 mcg	200 mcg	200 mcg
Selenium	55 mcg	65 mcg	75 mcg	75 mcg

Phytochemicals

We all marvel at the beauty of hillsides covered with wildflowers, at forests abundantly green, and relish the refreshing crunch of a fresh salad. Plants nurture the mind and body. It's a proven fact that green is the color that helps people feel the most serene. And it's also a fact that plants rich in phytochemicals carry many of the elements our bodies need to fight disease. Although many researchers don't classify phytochemicals as essential nutrients like vitamins and minerals, I do because they protect the body from inflammation, cancer, and other diseases. Phytochemicals promote good health; they come from plants, so that means fruits, vegetables, legumes, and grains are rich sources. (And a big plus is that they are not destroyed when the plants are cooked!)

These phytochemicals actually help plants fight diseases, and many scientists believe that they help our bodies do the same. We don't need phytochemicals, unlike vitamins and minerals, to literally stay alive, but they work synergistically with vitamins and minerals to promote good health and lower the risk of diseases such as cancer. Phytochemicals work like antioxidants, protecting cells from destruction and working to deactivate cancer-causing substances in the body. Research on the health effects of phytochemicals has increased exponentially during the past decade with hundreds of phytochemical-related articles published each year, in large part spurred on by what many view as the protective effects of fruits and vegetables.

A big plus for new moms is that phytochemicals work hard to balance hormones. Plus, they also help to combat the stress—both physical and emotional—of your new life. With a diet rich in these biologically active chemicals, you'll be far less vulnerable to stress-related illness. For you as a new mom, phytochemicals are the proverbial lifesaver, so I think of them as essential nutrients and emphasize them in every meal. I encourage you to eat as many phytochemical-rich fresh fruits and vegetables as you can every day so that your body has a constant infusion of nourishing, natural disease fighters.

While phytochemicals are found in our favorite fruits and vegetables, don't forget that nuts, whole grains, and soy products also come from plants, so they're rich in phytochemicals too. There are many different types of phytochemicals, some you've probably heard of, such as the flavonoids that are prevalent in many fruits and veggies, as well as green tea and various soy products and the lycopenes that are available in tomatoes. Others have less familiar names like lignans and isothio-cyanates. You don't need to know the complicated names to know that phytochem-icals are working for you whenever you eat fresh, unprocessed foods derived from plants.

Micronutrients and Your Hormones

Your hormones will never rage as wildly as they did during the last forty weeks of pregnancy. All the estrogen, progesterone, insulin, HCG, thyroid, and leptin in your body were working together to create the same baby fat they're going to help you lose in the next several weeks. Hormones also made you happy, sad, energetic, or lethargic, interested in sex or repulsed by it, and, yes, hungry or not. Just about every mood swing can be attributed to those chemical messengers that were work-ing overtime during your pregnancy. And now, they are affecting you just as strongly. The hormones themselves are not fully responsible for these highs and lows, however. Hormones are inextricably linked to natural chemicals in the brain called neurotransmitters—dopamine, serotonin, endorphins, epinephrine, and nor-epinephrine—that work with your hormones, and influence emotions, how you sleep, how much energy you have, and so on. Food has an impact on these neuro-transmitters, so by eating properly you have some control over your hormones.

It's a well-accepted fact that folic acid has a positive impact on alleviating de-pression because it causes serotonin levels in the brain to increase. Psychiatric pa-tients with depression have much higher rates of folic acid deficiency than the general public. As little as 200 micrograms a day was enough to relieve the depres-sion. That's easily attainable in a cup of cooked spinach or two oranges. Apply that to your life right now if you've got the baby blues. Attack that folic acid deficiency with a big spinach salad and add some mandarin orange slices and diced red bell peppers to it. Dress it with a raspberry vinagrette and sprinkle a few raisins on top for an added boost.

Or maybe you've felt that your brain's a little foggy; you're not as alert as you'd like to be. Eating protein allows the amino acid tyrosine to tell your brain to in-crease your body's production of dopamine, epinephrine, and norepinephrine. My shorthand for these neurotransmitters is "the happy hormones" because not only will they lift your spirits, they also will make you feel alert and energized. So when you need an energy boost, don't turn to sugar; instead, try the long-lasting effects of high-protein foods such as cheese, milk, tofu, meat, fish, poultry, and eggs. A tablespoon of reduced-fat peanut butter spread on apple slices makes a great mid-afternoon snack that activates the production of happy hormones.

When you're stressed, your body needs serotonin to produce a sense of calm, reduce pain, decrease appetite, and induce sleep. That's where complex carbohydrates come in—they release insulin into the bloodstream, and insulin clears amino acids out of the blood, except for tryptophan, which is converted to serotonin. The *Body After Baby* plan contains foods that influence neurotransmitters, so you'll feel much more in control of your hormone-induced emotions, moods, sleep patterns, and appetite.

When you enter the postpartum period your levels of estrogen and progesterone drop, slowly returning to the normal, prepregnancy levels, and your serotonin levels drop too. These lower levels can make you feel depressed and inhibit weight loss. That's the most important reason *not* to adopt a high-protein, carbohydrate-deprived diet during this period. Complex carbohydrates increase the brain's production of serotonin, thus elevating your mood.

Here's where I make chocolate lovers happy. Do you know that chocolate positively affects your mood? It causes your brain to release serotonin, so you quickly feel calmer after eating it. You can change your mood, relax, even fall asleep by eating a little chocolate before bed. I encourage my *Body After Baby* moms who like chocolate to enjoy some whenever the stress gets to you. Don't go overboard, but don't skimp either—how about twenty-three M&M's? That's all it took for Uma Thurman when she was stressed. Now, all of you fellow chocolate lovers, celebrate!

Are Herbs Safe During Breast-Feeding?

Many herbs have not been well studied, and of those that are, some are particularly dangerous during pregnancy, as they can cause miscarriage or other complications. I spoke with an expert on the subject, W. Kip Johnson, M.D., who specializes in preventive medicine, about the safety of herbs after the baby is born. Here's what he told me: "During the postpartum period, some herbs can have undesired effects. For example, sage can stop breast milk production, while fenugreek, fennel seed, blessed thistle, and alfalfa are galactagogues, which means that they stimulate breast milk production. Most herbs that are appropriate for an individual at times unrelated to pregnancy are also appropriate during the postpartum period—if the mother is not lactating. Again, consultation with a trusted health-care practitioner is advised and essential."

Dr. Johnson cautions new moms that the FDA does not regulate herbs. "However, in the natural-products industry, efforts are being made by many companies to improve the consistency and assure the quality of herbal products," he points out. "In Europe, the German Commission E, one of the most recognized authorities on herbal products and similar to the U.S. Food and Drug Administration, has produced monographs recommending the uses, dosages, warnings, and contraindications of many herbs. These Commission E monographs are used as references by many health professionals in the United States. So if you have specific herbs that you would like to use, ask your caregiver to research these monographs if he or she is not familiar with them."

For more information you can talk to your caregiver or to a natural products pharmacist, and also visit the site of the American Botanical Council, an organization that compiles information about herbs, at www.herbalgram.org.

The Bottom Line

Vitamins, minerals, and phytochemicals are the micronutrients that make a huge difference in your energy levels, your sleep patterns, and your postpregnancy weight loss. The healthiest and safest way to attain these is through the foods you eat—you can't overdose the way you can with over-the-counter supplements. Check with your health-care professional, but in most cases, if you follow the *Body After Baby* plan, you won't need additional supplements. Keep *Body After Baby* as a guide to the Super Foods that provide the essential micronutrients, and keep the following four facts in mind as you plan your meals:

1. Eat from the entire spectrum of color when it comes to fruits and vegetables. Think of a rainbow and choose from every hue. Dark leafy greens, red peppers and apples, orange and yellow citrus fruits, peaches and apricots, deep purple blueberries—the more colors the better.
2. Plant foods contain abundant phytochemicals that have great nutritive value, so indulge in as many plant-derived foods in their natural state whenever possible.
3. Remember the key antioxidants: beta-carotene, vitamins C and E, selenium, zinc, manganese, copper, and iron. Strive to incorporate many of these disease-

fighting compounds into your daily diet. You can't overdose on antioxidants if you're getting them from food.

4. Look for vitamin- and mineral-fortified food options when buying commercial products in the grocery store. A good example is calcium-fortified orange juice or vitamin-fortified whole-grain cereals. Every time you make this choice, you increase your intake of important nutrients.

jackie keller's 30-day
body after baby plan

THIS IS THE BIG CHAPTER—the *Body After Baby* plan. You're on your way to losing that excess baby weight and gaining a stronger, healthier body. You're going to be amazed at how much better and slimmer you feel each day. You'll have energy and you'll sleep soundly. You'll also be in great shape to take care of your wonderful baby.

Maybe you're reading this chapter first because you just want to know what the "diet" is like. That's okay! But please remember that this is not a diet book—in my mind, "diet" is a four-letter word. The *Body After Baby* plan is a great way to eat breakfast, lunch, dinner, and snacks for the rest of your life because the dishes are filled with lots of good, healthy, easy-to-fix food. If you haven't already done so, go back and read the other chapters because it's extremely important that you under-stand why this plan is designed as it is. When you know exactly why you're eating what you're eating, you'll understand all of the reasons that eating well is making you feel so good. Plus, after the first thirty days, you will have tasted dozens of great recipes and, when you understand the nutritional balance that provides the basis for the plan, you can adjust your meals to suit your personal preferences. The plan is flexible—you can schedule your snacks about two and a half to three hours after breakfast and lunch, or when the baby takes naps. You can have your evening snack as dessert with dinner, or you can save it for later. It's easy to make the plan work for you.

The Essential Movement Component

Each day of the plan features what I call a **Movement Focus.** I'll give you a new exercise that will help firm and tone parts of your body that have been stretched for nine months and that will work the muscles that you may not have used much recently. You're probably saying, "Yeah, right, Jackie. I barely have time to take a shower. I'm always with the baby, or I'm napping when she's asleep. When can I exercise?" At first, that's what a new mom's life feels like. Pressed for time. Zapped for energy. Chronically sleep-deprived. But I promise you can exercise and not take time away from your little one, the rest of your family, or from whatever precious sleep time you can find. In fact, the bonuses to the *Body After Baby* plan will be that you sleep more soundly, and when you're awake you'll have so much energy that you'll find more time each day to tackle what everyone else thinks is the impossible for a mom with a newborn.

To start off, before doing anything else, there's one exercise that I want you to do every day, whenever you think about it—while you're feeding the baby, brushing your teeth, paying bills, or doing the laundry: Kegels. The Kegel exercise is designed to strengthen and tighten the pelvic-floor muscles. Your cervix and vagina, not surprisingly, have been stretched considerably and your pelvic-floor muscles are soft and slack. Your cervix will firm up by itself in a week or so, but your pelvic floor needs some help from you—that's where Kegels can help. They tighten that pelvic floor quickly and painlessly. If you already know how to do a Kegel, start doing them as you read this. If you've never done a Kegel, here's how: First contract your anus (as if you were trying to prevent passing gas) and relax; then contract the urinary sphincter muscle (as if you were trying to stop urine flow) and relax; finally, contract your vaginal muscles, hold for five seconds (work up to ten if you can), and relax; then repeat the series. To really make the Kegels effective, build up to five contractions about ten times a day. In addition to strengthening and tightening your pelvic floor muscles, Kegels may speed up healing from an episiotomy, and will help avoid stress incontinence in the future.

Every mom needs daily exercise. How much and how soon after you give birth is a question for your health-care professional. The exercises in the *Body After*

Baby plan are designed to be gentle, but effective. However, as a precaution before beginning any new exercise program, show the plan to your health-care professional and ask for his or her input in case you have special postpartum needs. (Keep in mind if you experience any bleeding or blood in the lochia—the postpartum vaginal discharge, which is naturally blood-red during the first few days after pregnancy and changes to pink, then brown, then clear—you should stop exercising and consult your health-care professional for personalized advice.)

Once you've got the clearance, proceed carefully and be sure to follow these simple guidelines: (1) Make certain that your posture is never contorted when you are doing any exercise. Keep your body as relaxed as possible, trying to tense only the muscles you are working out. (2) Warm up for about five minutes before doing any sort of exercise. Marching in place is a great way, but you can walk on a treadmill, ride a stationary bike, or do anything else that gradually raises your body temperature. Studies have shown that stretching before your body temperature is elevated increases the risk of injury, so warm up first.

All the movements in the *Body After Baby* plan should be done in a slow and steady manner, and each day I've included **Today's Movement Plan** to remind you of which exercises to do. Do them at least once a day, or more often if you have time. Some of the stretches will feel so good that you'll find yourself doing them throughout the day to help reduce your stress.

Pregnancy and postnatal exercise specialist Rick Barke makes an important point: "You don't have to be afraid of exercising after giving birth. If you warm up, move carefully, and listen to your body, you'll find that exercise helps you to regain your strength, your energy, and restful sleep."

BREAST-FEEDING AND THE *BODY AFTER BABY* PLAN

The *Body After Baby* plan is for *all* moms, whether or not you're breast-feeding. The American Academy of Pediatrics recommends that you continue breast-feeding exclusively until your child is at least six months old and preferably for the entire first year of life. When you consider that new babies who are fed on demand will nurse anywhere from eight to twelve times a day, that's a lot of milk your body needs to produce. So you want a strong, healthy body. That's why the calorie count in the *Body After Baby* menu plan is for breast-feeding moms.

Health-care professionals are in agreement on the subject of breast-feeding.

When you have a new baby, it's the best thing you can do to protect your child's health. Breast-feeding provides optimal nutrition for your baby and provides protection from infections because your immunities are passed through to your child through your milk. Research shows that compared to bottle-fed infants a breast-fed baby will also suffer fewer colds, flu, and other respiratory illnesses, will have fewer sicknesses that require doctor visits, and is more likely to maintain a healthy weight later in life.

Of course, some moms can't nurse or choose not to nurse. If you are advised not to breast-feed for health reasons or you've made the decision not to nurse, your pediatrician will guide you through strengthening your child's immune system and keeping your infant healthy. But it's up to you to keep yourself strong and healthy, too, so you can take care of your baby. You need the *Body After Baby* plan just as much as a breast-feeding mom does. However, you don't need the additional 500 to 750 calories each day that producing breast milk demands. Depending on your height, weight, and activity level, you *do* need a minimum of 1,200 to 1,500 calories a day just to stay energized. Even though you don't need the extra calories, you absolutely need all the nutrients, so don't shortchange yourself. To accommodate your caloric requirement, there's a box on each day of the plan that tells you how to adapt each day's menu to suit your needs. To make it easy, I've adjusted portions on each day's menu and let you know what to do each day. If you get extra hungry from time to time, select an extra snack from the low-calorie "free" foods in the box below.

Just a reminder about the importance of water: It's important to drink at least 80 ounces of water each day—one cup every hour for ten hours. If you are breast-

low-calorie "free" foods

½ grapefruit	6 cauliflowerets	1 cup turnip
½ cup melon	½ cup celery	½ cup watercress
½ orange	½ large cucumber	1 cup low-sodium vegetable
1 peach	1 cup salad greens	broth
1 plum	½ cup mushrooms	1 cup low-sodium V8 or
½ cup strawberries	½ cup bell pepper	low-sodium tomato juice
1 scrambled egg white	1 cup radishes	
½ cup cabbage	1 medium tomato	

feeding it is imperative that you drink at least three quarts of water a day, or about two cups each hour. You will stay properly hydrated and your milk production will be abundant. Whether you're breast-feeding or not, don't try to drink sugary sodas or artificially-sweetened beverages as a substitute for plain water. Your body needs the purity and healing properties of simple, unadulterated water. If you'd like to squeeze the juice of orange, lemon, or lime into the water, enjoy it as a change of pace.

Stock Your Fridge and Pantry

Before you begin the *Body After Baby* plan, take a trip to the market to stock up on healthy ingredients. On page 330 I've provided a list of foods you'll need for the first ten days of the plan. The food you'll buy will be supergood for you—no unhealthy foods or empty calories. Instead, they will be loaded with nutrients and full of fresh flavor. If you're already home with baby and just don't feel like you can face the checkout stand yet, ask your husband, mom, sister, or any of those fabulous friends who asked how they can help to make the trip for you.

As a general rule, read packaged food labels carefully. Please remember to purchase products that contain less than 1 gram of trans fats, information you can find by reading the Nutrition Facts label on commercial food products. I discussed these harmful fats at length in chapter 2, but I want to remind you to be on the lookout for them. Also, avoid products whose ingredient list includes high-fructose corn syrup among the first few ingredients. High-fructose corn syrup contains no healthy nutrients and should be minimized in all diets. Those are rules I'm pretty rigid about. But I want to encourage you to relax and enjoy the meal plan and not obsess when it comes to ingredients. Consider these points:

- Buy fat-free dairy products and salad dressings whenever possible, but when your store doesn't carry something in a fat-free version, simply buy the product with the lowest fat content you can find.
- When you're shopping for greens to make a salad, try to select as many dark leafy greens as possible. A pale iceberg lettuce is great for its fiber and water content, but dark green romaine and red leaf lettuce have eight times more vitamin C than iceberg. So buy dark greens often and in generous amounts.
- I'm so lucky to live in California, where fruits and veggies are abundant year-round. That may not be the case for you, so select frozen versions if you can't

find fresh. A package of frozen mixed veggies is a great substitute and makes your life easier.

- You'll notice I recommend whole-grain products whenever possible. If you can't find whole-grain pastas or breads, ask your grocer to order them for you. In the meantime, make the recipe with the products that are available to you. All of the recipes are inherently healthy, so your progress won't be hampered. Whole grains offer you more nutrients and that's why I recommend them.

In addition, I recommend that you follow these straightforward and simple rules about beverages:

- Drink at least 8 ounces of water with each meal and no more than 8 ounces of fruit juice each day, unless specified in the meal plan for that day.
- Limit diet soda to no more than one 12-ounce serving daily. Eliminate all soda, if possible.
- If you're nursing, be sure to drink an additional 16 ounces of plain, pure water during each nursing session. I had one client who always kept a fresh 16-ounce bottle of water next to her nursing chair and made a point to finish it by the time baby was finished nursing. That was her way of making certain she was always getting enough water.
- You may have coffee and tea with caffeine in moderation—no more than one to two cups per day, in addition to the water. Avoid alcohol when breast-feeding. It contains empty calories and can disrupt your sleep.

Remember to consult your health-care professional before beginning any weight loss program and be sure to ask if you should be taking a multivitamin each day.

Let's Get Started!

There are three ten-day phases to the plan. Each one has a special, "super" focus.

Phase 1: **Super Easy**—This phase is super because no meal takes more than ten minutes to prepare and none of the recipes has more than ten ingredients. Each day's menu is designed to make your life super easy. The nutritious foods will help you sleep soundly and the simple exercises are gentle healing movements that are

easy to do anytime. For your first few days with a newborn, it's imperative that your daily routine is as basic as possible and that your food is as nutritious as it can be!

Phase 2: **Super Foods**—These meal plans are loaded with nutrients for maximum energy, and the high levels of antioxidants will speed your body's natural healing. Although none of the Phase 2 recipes require more than fifteen minutes to prepare, every ingredient will give you the boost you need for extra energy to devote to your baby, your spouse, your other kids, and—don't forget!—yourself. This complete nutrition will help you heal more rapidly after the birth process. The exercises will help to strengthen those muscles that have done double duty for forty long weeks, and they'll increase your stamina and endurance.

Phase 3: **Super Performance**—This ten-day phase is filled with high-performance foods and exercises that will make you feel strong and energetic. By your third week postpartum, it's time to focus on providing your body with nature's very best performance enhancers such as fish, berries, and whole-grain cereals. Eating right couldn't be more important, as it's a critical part of keeping your hormones working in the most favorable weight loss and energy-boosting mode. These menus are loaded with super performance meals—premium fuel for your busy days. You'll notice that you aren't craving as much sleep, your mind will be clearer, and you'll learn recipes that you can use for the rest of your life. The quick twenty-minute daily workout will help keep you in shape for the rest of your life.

If you are a vegetarian, all of the information I've provided applies to you—all that changes are the meals. The alternative fifteen-day *Body After Baby* vegetarian menu plan, which you can repeat, is in chapter 5. These menus are carefully planned to make sure that your macronutrients and micronutrients are balanced and your complete protein needs are met. Use the same movement plans that are listed in this chapter.

Day 1

I don't want you to have to think about anything but your baby and feeling stronger, so all the food you eat today is easy to prepare and full of flavor. Blueberries, whether they're fresh or frozen, are a Super Food that will help keep your mind clear! Like blueberries, peanut butter is one of the Super Foods you'll be eating throughout this plan because it has important nutrients that keep your system working at peak performance. If you prefer, you can substitute a different nut butter such as almond butter for the peanut butter. Save your Chocolate Chip Fondue dessert until just before bedtime. Chocolate stimulates the production of serotonin, which helps to naturally induce a sense of well-being, which in turn can lead to sounder sleep—what a wonderful treat! If you're not a chocolate lover, make a vanilla- or butterscotch-chip fondue for a healthy sweet. This fondue is one of Uma Thurman's favorite foods, and once you taste it, you'll know why.

BREAKFAST

1 poached egg (or you can have it prepared any other way, without additional fat)
1 slice whole-grain toast
1 tsp. trans fat–free light margarine or spread
½ cup blueberries

MORNING SNACK

½ large apple, sliced
¼ cup pumpkin seeds

LUNCH

¾ cup *Turkey Salad* (see recipe on page 314)
1 whole-wheat pita
¾ cup calcium-fortified orange juice (or other 100% fruit, calcium-fortified juice)

AFTERNOON SNACK

1 banana
1 Tbsp. all-natural, reduced-fat peanut butter
1 cup fat-free milk

DINNER

1 serving *Chicken Teriyaki* (see recipe on page 201)
½ cup *Spinach Pilaf* (see recipe on page 296)
As much as you want of dark leafy greens as a salad with tomatoes, cucumbers, and your favorite veggies. (Make colorful choices for the most beneficial nutrients.)
1 Tbsp. low-fat (less than 5 g fat/serving) or fat-free salad dressing

SNACK/DESSERT

3 Tbsp. *Chocolate Chip Fondue* (see recipe on page 205)
3 low-fat graham crackers

If You're Not Breast-Feeding

REDUCE:

Pumpkin seeds to 2 Tbsp. (1 oz.)
   at Morning Snack
Whole-wheat pita to ½ at Lunch
Peanut butter to ½ Tbsp.
   at Afternoon Snack
Chocolate Chip Fondue to 2 Tbsp.
   at Snack/Dessert
Graham crackers to 2
   at Snack/Dessert

ELIMINATE:

Orange juice at lunch

MOVEMENT FOCUS

Today your emphasis should be on relaxing whenever it's possible. Do a breathing exercise that is simple but refreshing: Start with five very slow deep breaths (inhale and exhale slowly just to slow yourself down). In a seated position, stretch your arms gently toward the ceiling, inhaling as you reach as high as you can. Hold for the count of three and lower your arms very slowly, exhaling. Repeat this three times. Repeat the set four times throughout the day.

Today's **Movement Focus** stretch is the very relaxing Upper Body Stretch, an exercise you'll do daily as often as you can, like your Kegels.

Upper Body Stretch

❋ While standing or seated in a chair, make certain your back is straight and your feet are planted firmly on the floor (or if you prefer, sit cross-legged on the floor).

❋ Reach up with your left arm toward the ceiling, stretching up and out from your left hip and tightening your abdominals.

❋ Reach as high as you can, hold the stretch for a few seconds, and relax.

❋ Repeat with the other arm. Do one set of ten repetitions (ten stretches with each arm).

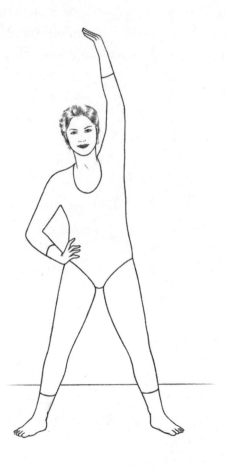

Day 2

Breakfast is always an easy-to-prepare meal on the *Body After Baby* plan. In addition to providing a super-start for each day, there are many health benefits associated with eating breakfast. Studies have shown that breakfast eaters are a third less likely to be obese and half as likely to have blood sugar problems. Also, eating breakfast helps regulate appetite levels throughout the day.

Today you'll have more delicious meals rich with fiber to keep your system working efficiently. Notice too that there are several Super Foods on the list: blueberries, spinach, and broccoli. The delicious dinner recipe today is Sautéed Fish Fillets with Lime—one of Susan Sarandon's favorites.

BREAKFAST

1 cup whole-grain breakfast cereal (use one with at least 6 g dietary fiber and protein/serving)
1 cup fat-free milk
¼ whole banana, sliced
½ cup blueberries

MORNING SNACK

1 orange
½ oz. pistachio nuts

LUNCH

1 *Ipanema Wrap* (see recipe on page 251)
1 ¼ cups *Spinach, Tomato, and Red-Onion Salad* (see recipe on page 300)
1 cup fat-free milk

AFTERNOON SNACK

½ cup *Power Snack Mix* (see recipe on page 279)

DINNER

5 oz. *Sautéed Fish Fillets with Lime* (see recipe on page 287)
½ cup baked yams
1 cup steamed broccoli

SNACK/DESSERT

12 animal crackers
1 cup vanilla fat-free yogurt

If You're Not Breast-Feeding

REDUCE:

Power Snack Mix to ¼ cup at Afternoon Snack
Animal crackers to 6 at Snack/Dessert
Vanilla fat-free yogurt to ½ cup at Snack/Dessert

ELIMINATE:

Pistachio nuts at Morning Snack

MOVEMENT FOCUS

Continue with your Upper Body Stretches and Kegels. Today, add a new Movement Focus: your abdominal muscles. (Yes, they're still there; they just need some attention to get stronger and firmer.) Here's a quick test to try before you start. Quite often, the longitudinal abdominal muscles separate toward the end of pregnancy; the medical term for this is *diastasis recti*. Don't let the terminology worry you. It is a perfectly normal condition—it's how your body made room for your baby to grow. To check for *diastasis recti* (or separation of your main abdominal muscle):

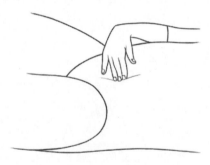

❀ Lie on your back with knees bent and feet flat on the floor or the bed.

❀ Slowly raise your head and shoulders, tightening your abdominal muscles.

❀ Keeping the muscles tight, put your index and middle fingers on your belly just below your belly button and press in slightly. You should feel a soft gap between hard muscle on either side as you move your fingers from side to side. You can gauge how well they are getting back into shape after childbirth by checking regularly (every couple of weeks) to see that the gap is closing up.

To begin strengthening your abdominals, try the Pelvic Tilt, another relaxing movement.

Pelvic Tilt

❀ Lie on your bed or on the floor on your back with your knees bent. Your arms can be at your sides, or gently folded over your ribs, as in the illustration.

❀ Breathe in slowly through your nose, then exhale through parted lips and draw in your abdominal muscles, pushing your back into the bed and tilting your pelvis.

❀ Hold for a count of four and gently relax.

❀ Do one set of three repetitions, or more if it feels comfortable.

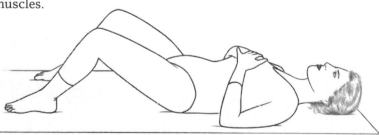

Day 3

The variety of food continues with lots of delicious vegetables and some wonderful fruit. Notice that the protein portions are small and the veggie portions are big. Today's menu also includes two great-for-you nuts, almonds and walnuts. They're loaded with healthy fats and oils, exactly what your body needs.

BREAKFAST

½ cup instant oatmeal, prepared according to package directions, substituting ½ cup unsweetened apple juice for water (about the amount that would fit in a medium-size coffee mug)

½ cup chopped apple, stirred into oatmeal for sweetening

1 cup fat-free milk

MORNING SNACK

4 Tbsp. dried fruit, such as raisins

1 oz. almonds

LUNCH

4 oz. *Shrimp Salad* (see recipe on page 289)

1 Tbsp. low-fat (less than 5 g fat/serving) or fat-free salad dressing

1 whole-wheat roll

1 reduced-fat string cheese

AFTERNOON SNACK

1 pear

1 oz. walnuts

DINNER

4 oz. *Roast Beef* (about the size of an audio cassette or a standard deck of playing cards) (see recipe on page 283)

½ medium-size (about 3 inches) corn on the cob

1 cup steamed or sautéed zucchini

As much as you want of dark leafy greens as a salad with tomatoes, cucumbers, and your favorite veggies. (Make colorful choices for the most beneficial nutrients.)

1 Tbsp. low-fat (less than 5 g fat/serving) or fat-free salad dressing

SNACK/DESSERT

½ cup reduced-fat chocolate ice cream

½ cup sliced fresh strawberries

If You're Not Breast-Feeding

REDUCE:

Almonds to ½ oz. at Morning Snack

Walnuts to ½ oz. at Afternoon Snack

Roast Beef to 3 oz. at Dinner (a little smaller than the size of an audio cassette or a standard deck of playing cards)

ELIMINATE:

String cheese at Lunch

MOVEMENT FOCUS

Continue with your Kegels, building up by extending the contraction time to ten seconds. You'll keep your **Movement Focus** on your tummy again today. This abdominal contraction replaces yesterday's exercise.

Abdominal Contraction

❋ Lie on your bed or on the floor with your knees bent and your feet flat.

❋ Exhale and tighten your abdominals while tilting your pelvis so that the hollow of your back flattens onto the bed or floor.

❋ Slide your left foot forward as far as you can without arching your back.

❋ Slide your foot back to the starting position.

❋ Repeat the movement with your right leg. Initially, your back may arch when your feet are only a few inches away. This is because your abdominal muscles have been weakened. As you get stronger, you'll be able to extend your leg farther, contracting your stomach muscles tightly while you continue to press your back to the floor.

❋ Repeat ten times with each leg.

TODAY'S MOVEMENT PLAN

Today's Movement Plan will list the movements to do each day. You may do them whenever you have time during your busy day. If you do the movements in one time period, do them in the order listed, so you progressively work the muscles in your body from your head to your toes. As days go by, I will add new movements to the list and replace others, so read the list each day.

Kegels: as often as you can, at least twice a day
Upper Body Stretch: as often as you can
Abdominal Contractions: ten repetitions with each leg

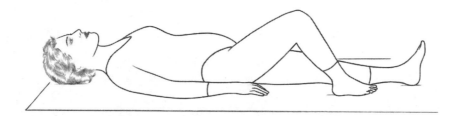

h.a.l.t.s. eating when you're not hungry

HERE'S a simple system you can use to analyze your urges to eat, since it's not always hunger that makes us want food. I've developed the **H.A.L.T.S.** system, as I've come to call it, to analyze "hunger" pangs. These pangs usually mean that you're either truly **H**ungry, or you're **A**ngry, **L**onely, **T**ired, or **S**tressed. So before you reach for food, think **H.A.L.T.S.** and ask yourself why you want it. When your children get older, you can help them to think about the reasons why they want to eat. Instead of "medicating" with food, there are other options. If you are **H**ungry, *truly* hungry: Eat a small handful of nuts. The healthy fats will satisfy you and provide some fast energy.

If you are **A**ngry and you think you want to eat: Write down your feelings first (many of my clients send their journal sheets to me, just so they know someone is reading them. You can too if you want to; just send your journal entries to me at jkeller@nutrifitonline.com), and if you still feel the need to eat, have a soothing carbohydrate in its purest form. Try half a baked potato or a piece of whole-grain bread. Add no fats such as butter or sour cream.

If you are **L**onely, *do not eat.* Write some of your thank-you notes. Call your best friend and cuddle your wonderful child! Food is never a cure for loneliness. Connecting with someone is!

If you are **T**ired, eat some water. Yes, *eat* some water. Dehydration causes fatigue, and the most satisfying way to ingest water is with food that is high in fluid content: Have some watermelon, an orange, or some cucumber slices.

If you are **S**tressed, stop what you are doing and pick up your baby and take a walk outside. Very often, just the change of scenery helps. A brief walk outside is refreshing, giving you a chance to think, slow down, and *not* eat. Eating when you're stressed will become a habit that's hard to break.

Day 4

Pasta (whole-wheat has a delicious flavor) for dinner tonight is a true comfort food, especially when the sauce is a simple marinara. When you shop for prepared pastas, look for whole-wheat versions, since they're more nutritious.

BREAKFAST

1 *Bran Raisin Muffin* (see recipe on
    page 195, or use small store-bought
    variety, if made with whole grains)
2 egg whites scrambled with
    1 whole egg
1 tsp. trans fat–free light margarine
    or spread
1 cup fat-free milk

MORNING SNACK

½ cup grapes

2 stalks celery

2 Tbsp. Neufchâtel light cream cheese

LUNCH

1½ cups *Grilled Chicken Caesar Salad*
   (see recipe on page 240)

1 Tbsp. low–fat (less than 5 g fat/serving)
   or fat-free salad dressing

AFTERNOON SNACK

1 Asian pear

1 oz. peanuts

DINNER

1½ cups store-bought chicken ravioli
   with marinara sauce

1 cup *Fragrant Kale* (see recipe on page 224)

SNACK/DESSERT

½ cup vanilla fat-free yogurt

½ cup blueberries

If You're Not Breast-Feeding

REDUCE:

Light cream cheese to 1 Tbsp.
   at Morning Snack

Peanuts to ½ oz. at Afternoon
   Snack/Dessert

Ravioli to 1 cup at Dinner

ELIMINATE:

Whole egg for Breakfast

MOVEMENT FOCUS

Today the **Movement Focus** is Foot Circles to help your circulation. Foot Circles will get your blood circulating to speed repair and recovery, since your blood carries oxygen that helps promote healing.

Foot Circles

❁ Lie with your legs straight and feet together.

❁ Briskly point and flex your feet, bending at the ankle for about thirty seconds.

❁ Move your feet apart slightly and circle each foot twenty times in each direction.

❁ Repeat as often as you'd like throughout the day. You can also do this while you're sitting in a chair.

TODAY'S MOVEMENT PLAN

Kegels: as often as you can, at least twice a day

Upper Body Stretch: as often as you can

Abdominal Contractions: ten repetitions with each leg

Foot Circles: twenty circles in each direction

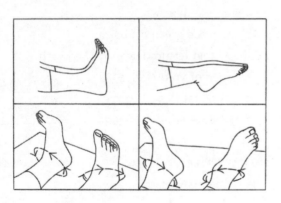

Day 5

Another day of deliciously easy meals. By now you might even know approximately how long your baby sleeps, so you can schedule your own in-the-house pleasures and give yourself some attention. Baby's naptime is a great opportunity to read the newspaper or take a leisurely bath.

By far my clients' favorite snack is the Peanut Butter Wrap (universally loved, and definitely at the top of Annabeth Gish's list). In addition to being truly delicious, it is one of the most nutrient-rich snacks you can choose. There is plenty of protein in the peanut butter and the light tofu, plus the banana offers vitamins and an extra boost of energy. And speaking of protein, cottage cheese is a great source of protein and calcium, a nutrient that is essential all through our lives, but especially when nursing.

BREAKFAST

1 *Peanut Butter Wrap* (see recipe on page 274)
¾ cup calcium-fortified orange juice (or other 100 percent fruit, calcium-fortified juice)

MORNING SNACK

1 cup fat-free cottage cheese
1 cup juice-packed fruit cocktail
or
1 cup cut-up fresh fruit salad
1 Tbsp. chopped walnuts

LUNCH

4 oz. deli-counter roast beef (about the size of an audio cassette or a standard deck of playing cards)
1 red bell pepper, cut into strips
½ cup baby carrots
1 oz. whole-grain pretzels
1 cup fat-free milk

AFTERNOON SNACK

1 apple
1 reduced-fat string cheese

DINNER

1 serving *Grilled Salmon with Jicama Orange Salsa* (see recipe on page 242)
½ cup cooked brown rice
1 cup steamed green beans
1 cup red leaf lettuce leaves topped with veggies of your choice
1 Tbsp. low-fat (less than 5 g fat/serving) or fat-free salad dressing

SNACK/DESSERT

2 Tbsp. semisweet chocolate chips

If You're Not Breast-Feeding

REDUCE:
Cottage cheese to ½ cup at Morning Snack
Fruit cocktail to ½ cup at Morning Snack
Grilled Salmon with Jicama Orange Salsa to 4 oz. at Dinner
Semisweet chocolate chips at Snack/Dessert to 1 Tbsp. (and savor each one!)

MOVEMENT FOCUS

Today's **Movement Focus** is the Shoulder Shrug, which concentrates on the muscles that control your posture. The Shoulder Shrug is a great way to relax and start working on improving your posture.

Shoulder Shrug

❋ First, see how you're standing in the mirror.

❋ Tighten your tummy muscles and lift your shoulders up toward your ears, hold for 10 seconds, and release.

❋ Tighten your stomach again and pull your shoulders down, hold for ten seconds, and release.

❋ Repeat the entire movement ten times. You can do this several times a day until you become adjusted to standing up very straight. You'll soon notice that your neck is stronger and your stomach looks flatter, and you'll be doing a better job of supporting your entire body.

TODAY'S MOVEMENT PLAN

Kegels: as often as you can, at least twice a day

Upper Body Stretch: as often as you can

Abdominal Contractions: ten repetitions with each leg

Shoulder Shrug: ten times, as often as you can

Foot Circles: twenty circles in each direction

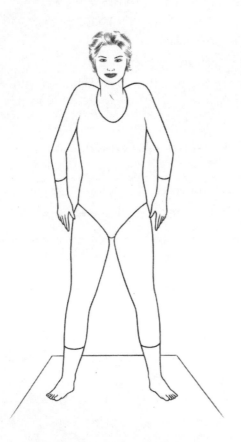

Day 6

Pork chops tonight! You'll find that pork is a low-fat alternative to beef and truly delicious. I like to serve it because it's high in protein, zinc, and potassium, and it's very high in the antioxidant selenium.

Are you finding ways to pamper yourself? Try taking some time out to give yourself a pedicure and then use a luxurious lotion on your feet and legs. You won't be as overly sensitive to fragrance as you may have been when you were pregnant, so there won't be a problem using your favorite scented lotion.

BREAKFAST

2 slices whole-grain bread, toasted
2 tsp. all-fruit preserves or trans fat–free
    light margarine or spread
½ grapefruit
1 mini Baby Bonbel light cheese

MORNING SNACK

½ cup fat-free cottage cheese
2 cups watermelon cubes

LUNCH

1 serving *Tomato Tuna Salad* (see recipe
    on page 310) topped with 2 Tbsp.
    wheat germ

AFTERNOON SNACK

2 oz. roasted soy nuts

¾ cup calcium-fortified orange juice
    (or other 100 percent fruit, calcium-
    fortified juice)

DINNER

1 serving *Hickory-Baked Pork Chops* (see
    recipe on page 246)
½ cup sweet potato, boiled and mashed
1 cup steamed green beans

SNACK/DESSERT

¼ cup *Piña Colada Dip* (see recipe on
    page 276)
1 banana

If You're Not Breast-Feeding

REDUCE:

Bread to 1 slice for Breakfast
Margarine, spread, or preserves to 1 tsp.
    for Breakfast
Wheat germ to 1 Tbsp. for Lunch
Hickory-Baked Pork Chop to 4 oz.
    for Dinner

MOVEMENT FOCUS

In addition to your relaxing daily stretches, the Kegels, and the other exercises you've learned, today you will add another important stretch—the Chest Stretch, which emphasizes your chest and pectoral muscles.

Chest Stretch

❋ Sit facing the back of a straight-backed chair with your legs straddling the seat.

❋ With your back straight, bring your arms behind you until you can loosely intertwine your fingers.

❋ Gently lift your arms and hands up while keeping your shoulders back and down.

❋ Hold the stretch for thirty seconds. You will feel the stretch across your chest. This is an especially good exercise if your breasts are feeling heavy.

❋ Do one set of three repetitions.

TODAY'S MOVEMENT PLAN

Kegels: as often as you can, at least twice a day

Upper Body Stretch: as often as you can

Abdominal Contractions: ten repetitions with each leg

Shoulder Shrug: ten times, as often as you can

Chest Stretch: three repetitions, anytime, but especially if your breasts feel heavy

Foot Circles: twenty circles in each direction

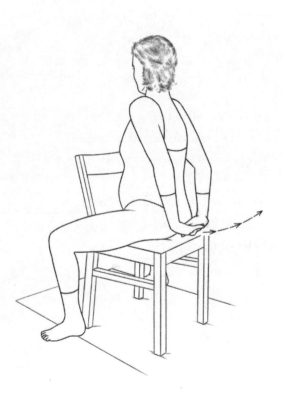

Day 7

Can you believe a week has passed already! I know you're feeling more energetic by now because the Super Foods are at work. Your mind is clearer and all the nutrients in your food are helping to speed the ongoing healing process.

Tonight's flavorful dinner feast is Seafood Fajitas. Actress/model Tia Carrere always requested Seafood Fajitas when she was one of our clients. They are light but filling, and so easy to prepare—it takes less than ten minutes and you've got a delicious meal.

BREAKFAST

1 *Cheese Omelet* (see recipe on page 197)
½ whole-grain English muffin
1 whole orange, cut into wedges

MORNING SNACK

1 grilled turkey sausage
1 apple

LUNCH

1 *Grilled Turkey Breast Sandwich* (see recipe on page 243)
1 cup assorted veggie sticks, such as celery, jicama, radishes, baby carrots

AFTERNOON SNACK

½ cup whole-grain peanut butter–filled pretzels

DINNER

6 oz. *Seafood Fajitas* (see recipe on page 289)
1 cup sliced summer squash
1 cup *Tomato, Mozzarella, and Basil Salad* (see recipe on page 311)

SNACK/DESSERT

One 4-inch slice *Angel Food Cake* (see recipe on page 180)
½ cup sliced strawberries

If You're Not Breast-Feeding

REDUCE:

Peanut butter-filled pretzels to ¼ cup at Afternoon Snack
Seafood Fajitas to 4 oz. at Dinner
Angel Food Cake to 2-inch slice at Snack/Dessert

ELIMINATE:

Turkey sausage at Morning Snack

MOVEMENT FOCUS

We're going to shift the **Movement Focus** to your shoulders with the Shoulder Roll. After you do your other daily movements, concentrate on relieving some of the tension that comes along with being a new mom.

Shoulder Roll

❋ Circle your right shoulder backward, then your left shoulder, then both.

❋ Repeat ten times, breathing easily and keeping your shoulders down and relaxed.

❋ Now reverse the motions, first rolling each shoulder forward, then both shoulders forward.

❋ Repeat ten times. You can do this exercise standing or sitting. Do it as frequently throughout the day as you can. Focus as you do each movement, and you'll feel renewed after each set.

TODAY'S MOVEMENT PLAN

Kegels: as often as you can, at least twice a day

Upper Body Stretch: as often as you can

Abdominal Contractions: ten repetitions with each leg

Shoulder Shrug: ten times, as often as you can

Shoulder Roll: ten times, as often as you can

Chest Stretch: three repetitions, anytime, but especially if your breasts feel heavy

Foot Circles: twenty circles in each direction

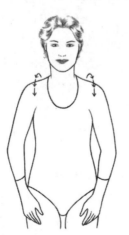
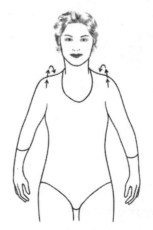

Day 8

You're into the second week of the program and it is time to add some new tastes and different textures. The *Body After Baby* recipes are suitable for the whole family, so you don't cook differently for everyone else just because you're losing weight. I've kept everything very simple, so the prep time for any meal is less than ten minutes. Today's menu is filled with fruits and vegetables, and they're all delicious. You'll notice that breakfast includes a serving of blackstrap molasses, which is a great source of calcium, iron, magnesium, potassium, copper, and manganese. It's a wonderfully nutritious food. If you don't care to eat it "straight," you can baste your meat loaf with the molasses instead. Also, some people prefer to eat ¼ cup of dried plums (prunes) instead of drinking prune juice—I leave it up to you. Either way will provide you with an excellent source of vitamin A, which the body synthesizes from beta-carotene in the fruit. Rich in bone-strengthening potassium, prunes provide plenty of fiber and are quite delicious.

Today you'll make a pot-full of delicious Vegetable Barley Soup. This recipe makes four servings, or you can double it and make eight so family and friends can share it with you. Freeze it in 1-cup containers and you'll enjoy it again on Day 11 and Day 13.

BREAKFAST

1 cup prune juice or 1 Tbsp. blackstrap molasses

½ cup *Couscous with Raisins and Dates* (see recipe on page 215)

1 cup fat-free milk

MORNING SNACK

½ cup fruit-flavored fat-free yogurt

LUNCH

¾ cup *Chicken Salad* (see recipe on page 199)

1 whole-wheat roll

½ cup grapes

AFTERNOON SNACK

1 cup raw vegetable sticks

2 Tbsp. *Creamy Herb Dressing* (see recipe on page 216)

DINNER

1 cup *Vegetable Barley Soup* (see recipe on page 317)

4 oz. *Vegetable-Stuffed Turkey Roll* (see recipe on page 318)

½ medium baked potato

2 cups cooked fresh spinach

SNACK/DESSERT

½ cup vanilla fat-free frozen yogurt topped with ½ cup frozen cherries

If You're Not Breast-Feeding

REDUCE:

Chicken Salad to ½ cup at Lunch

Whole-wheat roll to ½ roll at Lunch

Vegetable Barley Soup to ½ cup at Dinner

Vanilla fat-free frozen yogurt to ¼ cup at
    Snack/Dessert

MOVEMENT FOCUS

Today, the **Movement Focus** adds another stretch to your workout, the Neck Stretch. Do this stretch daily along with your Kegels, ankle circles, and shoulder rolls as many times as you can each day.

Neck Stretch

❀ Sitting cross-legged or in a straight-backeded chair, you're going to pull yourself up straight and tall.

❀ With your left arm, reach up and over the top of your head until your forefinger and middle finger touch your ear. Your right arm should be hanging loosely at your side with your wrist flexed and your palm down.

❀ Very gently pull your head toward your left shoulder. Do not strain, but feel the gentle stretch on the right side of your neck.

❀ Switch arms and put your right arm over your head. Gently pull your head toward your right shoulder. Hold the stretch to allow your muscles time to lengthen and relax.

❀ Do one set of five repetitions on each side, holding each stretch for the count of twenty.

TODAY'S MOVEMENT PLAN

Kegels: as often as you can, at least twice
    a day

Upper Body Stretch: as often as you can

Abdominal Contractions: ten repetitions
    with each leg

Shoulder Shrug: ten repetitions, as often
    as you can

Shoulder Roll: ten repetitions, as often as
    you can

Chest Stretch: three repetitions, anytime,
    but especially if your breasts feel heavy

Neck Stretch: five repetitions, as often as
    you can

Foot Circles: twenty circles in each
    direction

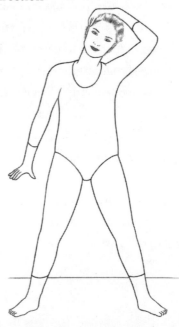

Day 9

Today you'll make your own delicious smoothie for a Morning Snack. The Wild Berry Smoothie was Uma Thurman's favorite when she was slimming down after childbirth, and before she knew it she was fit enough to *Kill Bill*. I'm also including a couple of recipes that each can be prepared in less than ten minutes. By now you've established a routine with the baby, so you know when you have time to cook.

Are you ready for a trip to the market? It's about time to restock! Schedule your trip to coincide with baby's nap, and let your husband, mom, or friend take care of your baby while you're gone. And if you're not up to shopping yet, delegate the job. Your new shopping list is on page 335.

BREAKFAST

2 Tbsp. wheat germ sprinkled on
   ¾ cup shredded-wheat squares
   (see note below)
1 cup fat-free milk

MORNING SNACK

5 oz. *Wild Berry Smoothie* (see recipe on page 322). Note: If you prefer, you can put 1 Tbsp. of wheat germ in your smoothie and reduce the amount in your breakfast meal.

LUNCH

1½ rolls *Lasagna Roll-ups* (see recipe on page 253)
As much as you want of romaine lettuce salad with tomatoes, cucumbers, and your favorite veggies. (Choose dark greens and other colorful vegetables for nutrient impact.)
1 Tbsp. low-fat (less than 5 g fat/serving) or fat-free salad dressing

AFTERNOON SNACK

2 oz. roasted soy nuts
¾ cup calcium-fortified orange juice (or other 100 percent fruit, calcium-fortified juice)

DINNER

1¼ cups *Spinach, Tomato, and Red-Onion Salad* (see recipe on page 300)
5 oz. *Lemon Basil Chicken* (see recipe on page 255)
½ cup *Lemon Rice* (see recipe on page 257)
½ cup cooked carrots

SNACK/DESSERT

1 store-bought biscotti
1 cup fat-free milk

If You're Not Breast-Feeding

REDUCE:

Lasagna Roll-ups to 1 roll at Lunch

Soy nuts to 1 oz. at Afternoon Snack

Lemon Basil Chicken to 4 oz. at Dinner

ELIMINATE:

Orange juice at Afternoon Snack

MOVEMENT FOCUS

Today's **Movement Focus** adds a lower body stretch to your daily routine. This is a great stretch to do at the end of your workouts.

Leg Stretch

❀ Sit on the edge of your chair (for safety's sake, no wheels or casters on your chair, please) with your right leg straight out in front of you and your left foot planted firmly on the ground.

❀ Reach down and hold the toes on your right foot, bending your right knee as needed, so it's easy to reach your toes.

❀ Now, slowly and gently, straighten your right leg while holding those toes. Maintain the stretch for ten seconds.

❀ Repeat with your left leg. Do one set of five repetitions with each leg.

TODAY'S MOVEMENT PLAN

Kegels: as often as you can, at least twice a day

Upper Body Stretch: as often as you can

Abdominal Contractions: ten repetitions with each leg

Shoulder Shrug: ten repetitions, as often as you can

Shoulder Roll: ten repetitions, as often as you can

Neck Stretch: five repetitions, as often as you can

Chest Stretch: three repetitions, anytime, but especially if your breasts feel heavy

Foot Circles: twenty circles in each direction as often as you can

Leg Stretch: five repetitions with each leg

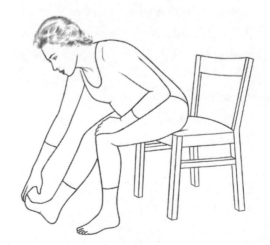

Day 10

This is the last day of Phase 1 of the *Body After Baby* plan. I'm sure by now you are feeling bursts of energy that you haven't experienced in months! And get on the scale today, because you're going to see tremendous progress. But after you weigh yourself, put that scale away and don't use it again until the end of Phase 2.

Throughout Phase 2, if you need help sleeping, revisit the desserts in Phase 1, which were designed to help you sleep more soundly. Tia Carrere loved the Peanut Butter–Hot Fudge Dip you'll have tonight. It will help you to sleep well until baby calls.

BREAKFAST

1 cup fat-free milk

1 small whole-wheat bagel

2 oz. fat-free cream cheese or 1 oz. Neufchâtel light cream cheese

2 cups fresh strawberries

MORNING SNACK

½ cup grapefruit

2 squares *Spinach, Cheese, and Mushroom Bake* (see recipe on page 298) with 2 Tbsp. wheat germ added into recipe before baking

LUNCH

1 serving *Egg Salad* (see recipe on page 219)

6 whole-grain crackers

1 cup cucumber and tomato slices

¾ cup calcium-fortified orange juice (or other 100 percent fruit, calcium-fortified juice)

AFTERNOON SNACK

1 cup *Greek Feta Salad* (see recipe on page 236)

1 banana

DINNER

1 serving *Baked Turkey Dijon* (see recipe on page 185)

½ cup brown or wild rice

½ cup mushrooms, sautéed in 1 tsp. extra-virgin olive oil

SNACK/DESSERT

2 Tbsp. *Peanut Butter–Hot Fudge Dip* (see recipe on page 273)

2 low-fat graham crackers

If You're Not Breast-Feeding

REDUCE:

Bagel to ½ for Breakfast

Fat-free cream cheese to 1 oz.; or Neufchâtel light cream cheese to ½ oz.
for Breakfast

Spinach, Cheese, and Mushroom Bake to
1 square for Morning Snack

Peanut Butter–Hot Fudge Dip to 1 Tbsp. for
Snack/Dessert

ELIMINATE:

Banana at Afternoon Snack

MOVEMENT FOCUS

Today's **Movement Focus** is the first aero-
bic component of your 30-day plan. And it's
simple: March in Place for a minimum of
three minutes. If you can, march vigorously
for five minutes, slow down for one minute, then vigorously for three minutes and
slow down for one minute, then rest. You can
march while you're watching the news or talking on the phone. You can do it holding the
baby or not. Whenever you can do it, do it.

TODAY'S MOVEMENT PLAN

As we enter Phase 2 of the plan, let's review
the movements you are doing now. From
today forward, if you do the exercises con-
secutively, warm up before the other movements with a March in Place, then warm

down with March in Place and the Leg
Stretch.

Kegels: as often as you can, at least twice
a day

March in Place: three minutes

Shoulder Roll: ten repetitions, as often
as you can

Neck Stretch: five repetitions, as often as
you can

Abdominal Contractions: ten repetitions
with each leg

Chest Stretch: three repetitions, anytime,
but especially if your breasts feel heavy

Foot Circles: twenty circles in each
direction

March in Place: seven minutes

Leg Stretch: five repetitions with each leg

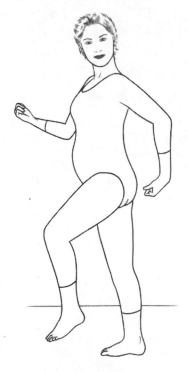

h.a.l.t.s.

BEFORE we move to Phase 2, let's revisit the **H.A.L.T.S.** system to help you quell any urges you may be having to overeat.

Hungry? Try ½ peanut butter sandwich on whole-grain bread or ½ peanut butter lavosh wrap; the healthy fat in peanut butter will calm those hunger pangs and tide you over until your next meal or snack.

Angry? Write in your journal about your feelings. And once you're feeling calmer, try to confront the problem head-on. Talking to your partner is your best place to start, even if he or she is not the source of the problem.

Lonely? Drink some water with lemon or lime juice and call a friend on the phone—immediately! Don't eat when you're lonely; instead, cure the "alone-ness."

Tired? Drink some water and eat some water—fruit and water are your greatest hydrators. Have a cool, refreshing glass of water and then slice a peach into a bowl and sprinkle 2 tablespoons of granola on top. The water will make you feel great and the healthy carbs will energize you.

Stressed? Use this progressive relaxation technique: Close your eyes, and slowly tense and then relax each part of your body, first your neck, then your shoulders, arms, and fingers; next, concentrate on your midsection/abdominal muscles, then your legs, feet, and toes. Each time you envision yourself getting more relaxed. When you've finished, breathe in deeply and very slowly exhale to release that tension.

Day 11

This is the first day of your Super Foods phase. You've been eating Super Foods since Day 1, but now I've added Super Foods to each meal, to make certain that your nutrient levels prepare your body for increasing activity each day. In Phase 2 you'll find that your energy levels are very high and so are your spirits. Speaking of spirits, Bryce Dallas Howard (the movie-star daughter of producer/director Ron Howard) really enjoyed the *Chicken with Creamy Herb Sauce* when she was filming the movie *The Village*.

BREAKFAST

½ grapefruit

3-inch square *Blueberry Lemon Coffee Cake* (see recipe on page 193)

1 cup fruit-flavored fat-free yogurt

MORNING SNACK

1 fresh peach

1 cup fat-free milk

LUNCH

2 cups *Pasta with White Beans* (see recipe on page 270)

As much as you want of dark leafy greens as a salad with tomatoes, cucumbers, and your favorite veggies. (Make colorful choices for the most beneficial nutrients.)

1 Tbsp. low-fat (less than 5 g fat/serving) or fat-free salad dressing

AFTERNOON SNACK

¼ cup *Artichoke Dip* (see recipe on page 181)

1 cup baby carrots

DINNER

1 cup *Vegetable Barley Soup* (defrost frozen portion you prepared on Day 8)

1 serving *Chicken with Creamy Herb Sauce* (see recipe on page 202)

1 cup brown rice

1 cup cooked spinach

SNACK/DESSERT

1 (4-oz.) cup store-bought, sugar-free pudding (any flavor)

2 plums

If You're Not Breast-Feeding

REDUCE:

Pasta with White Beans to 1 cup at Lunch

Chicken with Creamy Herb Sauce to 3 oz. at Dinner

Brown rice to ½ cup at Dinner

MOVEMENT FOCUS

Today's **Movement Focus** is on your abdominals, working toward a trimmer tummy. You'll add Reach and Crunch, an effective and easier alternative to sit-ups, after your Abdominal Contractions.

Reach and Crunch

❋ Lie on the floor with your knees bent and your feet flat on the floor.

❋ Tilt your pelvis, pulling in your abdominals, so that your back is flat on the floor. Support your head with your right hand.

❋ Bring your left shoulder (not just your arm) off the ground, curling up as you reach toward your right knee. Exhale as you lift, and hold the reach for the count of three before slowly lowering your body.

❋ Repeat with the other arm, reaching in the opposite direction. As you get stronger, you'll be able to roll up farther, but work up to it slowly.

❋ Start with one set of five repetitions on each side.

TODAY'S MOVEMENT PLAN

Kegels: as often as you can, at least twice a day

March in Place: three minutes

Shoulder Roll: ten repetitions, as often as you can

Neck Stretch: five repetitions, as often as you can

Abdominal Contractions: ten repetitions with each leg

Reach and Crunch: five repetitions on each side

Chest Stretch: three repetitions, anytime, but especially if your breasts feel heavy

Foot Circles: twenty circles in each direction

March in Place: seven minutes

Leg Stretch: five repetitions with each leg

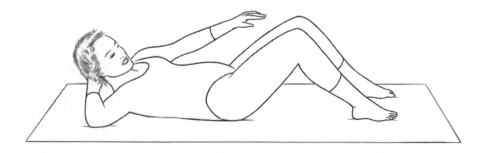

Day 12

Today's menu contains vegetarian favorites even meat lovers will enjoy. The salsa, *Eggless Egg Salad*, and pancakes were on menus provided for Charlize Theron, who rarely eats any type of animal-source foods.

Also on the menu today is *Fragrant Lentil Soup*. It's wonderfully rich with fiber, so a 2-cup serving is very filling. The recipe serves six, so freeze any leftovers in 1-cup containers so you can savor it again on Day 14 or when you need a healthy, filling snack.

BREAKFAST

1 cup prune juice, ¼ cup prunes,
    or 1 Tbsp. blackstrap molasses
4 *Blueberry Whole-Wheat Pancakes*
    (see recipe on page 194)
2 scrambled egg whites

MORNING SNACK

1 cup apple slices with peel
½ cup vanilla fat-free yogurt

LUNCH

1 cup *Eggless Egg Salad* (see recipe on page 220) as a sandwich on
    2 slices whole-wheat bread, toasted, with
    1 whole tomato, cut into wedges, and
    1 cup romaine or red-leaf lettuce leaves

AFTERNOON SNACK

1 cup jicama sticks
¼ cup *Black Bean Salsa* (see recipe on page 190)

DINNER

2 cups *Fragrant Lentil Soup* (see recipe on page 225)
1 serving *Oriental Red Snapper* (see recipe on page 265)
½ cup *Wild Rice Pilaf* (see recipe on page 323), or substitute ½ cup wild
    or brown rice
1 cup steamed broccoli

SNACK/DESSERT

2-inch square *Chocolate Chip Spice Cake* (see recipe on page 206), or
2 small store-bought, low-fat cookies

If You're Not Breast-Feeding

REDUCE:

Blueberry Whole-Wheat Pancakes to 2 for Breakfast
Whole-wheat bread to 1 slice for Lunch
Fragrant Lentil Soup to 1 cup for Dinner
Oriental Red Snapper to 4 oz. for Dinner

MOVEMENT FOCUS

Your **Movement Focus** today targets your waist. The Waist Trimmer also works your oblique muscles.

Waist Trimmer

❋ Lie on the floor with your knees bent slightly and your feet flat on the floor.

❋ Tilt your pelvis up, pressing your back to the floor while contracting your abdominals.

❋ Slide your left hand down toward your left foot, bending to the side at the waist. (Your head will naturally lift off the floor as you slide your arm down, alongside your body.)

❋ Count to three before returning to the starting position, then reach down your right side with your right hand.

❋ Do one set of five repetitions on each side.

TODAY'S MOVEMENT PLAN

Kegels: as often as you can, at least twice a day

March in Place: three minutes

Shoulder Roll: ten repetitions, as often as you can

Neck Stretch: five repetitions, as often as you can

Abdominal Contractions: ten repetitions with each leg

Reach and Crunch: five repetitions on each side

Waist Trimmer: five repetitions each side

Chest Stretch: three repetitions, anytime, but especially if your breasts feel heavy

Foot Circles: twenty circles in each direction

March in Place: seven minutes

Leg Stretch: five repetitions with each leg

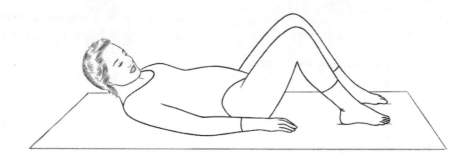

Day 13

I've added several new recipes for you to try; none are time-consuming, but they'll provide wonderful variety to your family fare.

Tomorrow will be two weeks since you began the program. Consider planning ahead and making an arrangement with your husband or a friend so you can have time to pamper yourself. Choose something that would be fun for you, something that feels special—even if it's a stroll in the park or in a museum for an hour.

BREAKFAST

1 cup cantaloupe melon cubes

1 whole-wheat bagel

1 Tbsp. all-natural, reduced-fat peanut butter

MORNING SNACK

½ cup grapes

1 cup fat-free milk, or 1 cube Laughing Cow light cheese

LUNCH

2-inch square *Vegetarian Enchilada Casserole* (see recipe on page 320) with 2 Tbsp. wheat germ mixed into casserole filling

As much as you want of dark leafy greens as a salad with tomatoes, cucumbers, and your favorite veggies. (Make colorful choices for the most beneficial nutrients.)

1 Tbsp. *Honey Balsamic Vinaigrette Dressing* (see recipe on page 249)

AFTERNOON SNACK

¼ cup *Spinach and Chive Dip* (see recipe on page 295) with

1 cup jicama or other veggie sticks

DINNER

1 cup *Vegetable Barley Soup* (defrost a frozen portion you prepared on Day 8)

1¼ cups *Oriental Beef with Peppers* (see recipe on page 264)

½ cup brown rice

SNACK/DESSERT

1 nectarine

1 cup fat-free frozen yogurt, your favorite flavor

If You're Not Breast-Feeding

REDUCE:

Bagel to ½ for Breakfast

Peanut butter to ½ Tbsp. for Breakfast

Spinach and Chive Dip to 2 Tbsp. for Afternoon Snack

Oriental Beef with Peppers to 1 cup for Dinner

Frozen yogurt to ½ cup for Snack/Dessert

MOVEMENT FOCUS

Today's **Movement Focus** movements are Wall Push-ups, which work the pectoral muscles of your chest.

Wall Push-ups

❋ Stand slightly more than arm's length from a wall, facing it, with feet slightly more than shoulder-width apart.

❋ Place your hands flat against the wall at shoulder height, with your fingers pointed straight up toward the ceiling.

❋ As you bend your elbows, press your chest toward the wall.

❋ Bring your chest as close to the wall as possible, then push back until your arms are straight again. Make sure you keep your back straight and heels on the ground.

❋ Do one set of ten repetitions.

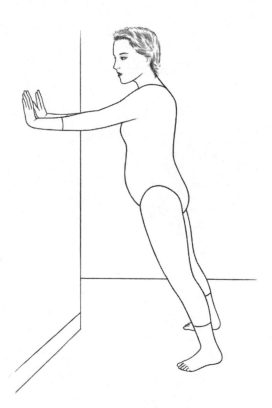
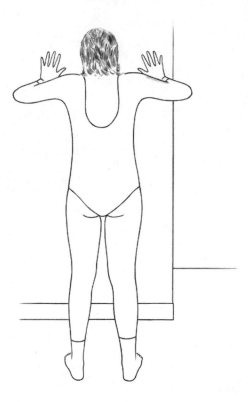

TODAY'S MOVEMENT PLAN

Kegels: as often as you can, at least twice a day

March in Place: three minutes

Shoulder Roll: ten repetitions, as often as you can

Neck Stretch: five repetitions, as often as you can

Reach and Crunch: five repetitions on each side

Waist Trimmer: five repetitions each side

Wall Push-ups: ten repetitions

Chest Stretch: three repetitions, anytime, but especially if your breasts feel heavy

March in Place: eight minutes

Leg Stretch: five repetitions with each leg

Day 14

You've been on the program for two weeks! Congratulations. Why not reward yourself with some lovely flowers, or better yet, a small perennial plant that blooms annually. Every year when it blooms you'll be reminded of the joy you feel now after the birth of your child. When each of our children were born, we planted a very small fruit tree—a seedling. The gorgeous flowers of "her" peach tree remind me of our daughter Alexandra's delicate beauty. We planted a plum tree for our son, Adam, and it bears the sweetest, juiciest Santa Rosa plums imaginable. The fruit is wonderful, just like he is.

More Super Foods are included today: chiles, peppers, and fresh strawberries. Enjoy!

BREAKFAST

1 Tbsp. blackstrap molasses
1 *Spanish Omelet* (see recipe on page 292)
1 slice whole-wheat bread, toasted
1 Tbsp. all-fruit preserves

MORNING SNACK

1 orange
½ cup fat-free cottage cheese

LUNCH

1½ cups *Fragrant Lentil Soup* (defrost a frozen portion you prepared on Day 12)

6 whole-grain crackers
1 cup celery sticks
1 oz. reduced-fat cheddar cheese

AFTERNOON SNACK

1 cup fat-free milk
1 piece *Cocoa Fruit Nougats* (see recipe on page 212)

DINNER

1 serving *Pork Kabobs* (see recipe on page 278)
½ cup whole-wheat couscous fluffed with 2 Tbsp. wheat germ
1 cup steamed green beans

SNACK/DESSERT

6 wedges *Dessert Nachos* (see recipe on page 218)

If You're Not Breast-Feeding

REDUCE:

Fragrant Lentil Soup to 1 cup for Lunch
Reduced-fat cheddar cheese to ½ oz. for Lunch
Pork Kabobs to 4 oz. for Dinner
Wheat germ to 1 Tbsp. for Dinner
Dessert Nachos to 4 wedges for Snack/Dessert

MOVEMENT FOCUS

Today's **Movement Focus** is Shoulder Blade Squeeze, which works the upper back and rear deltoid area.

Shoulder Blade Squeeze

❋ Stand straight with your right leg forward and slightly bent at the knee.

❋ Reach straight forward with your left arm, then in a nice clean movement, pull your arm back, pinching your shoulder blades together. Keep your elbow high and shoulders down.

❋ Repeat with your right arm, left leg forward.

❋ Do one set of ten repetitions on each side.

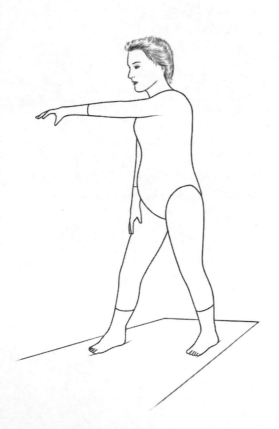
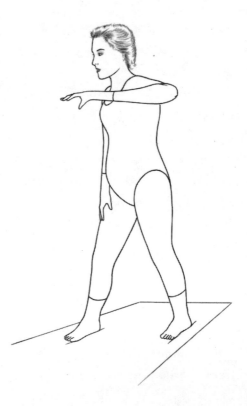

TODAY'S MOVEMENT PLAN

Kegels: as often as you can, at least twice
a day

March in Place: three minutes

Shoulder Roll: ten repetitions, as often as
you can

Neck Stretch: five repetitions, as often
as you can

Reach and Crunch: five repetitions on
each side

Waist Trimmer: five repetitions each side

Wall Push-ups: ten repetitions

Shoulder Blade Squeeze: ten repetitions
on each side

Chest Stretch: three repetitions, anytime,
but especially if your breasts feel heavy

March in Place: eight minutes

Leg Stretch: five repetitions with each leg

Day 15

Now that you're halfway through Phase 2, you should be feeling the benefits kick in, just as I've promised. Your body is properly nourished, and you're feeling energized. Today we add Crispy Baked Cod for dinner, rich with protein, to sustain your energy needs.

BREAKFAST

1 cup *Banana and Orange Oatmeal* (see recipe on page 187)

1 cup fat-free milk

MORNING SNACK

1 pear

1 oz. peanut butter–filled whole-grain pretzels

LUNCH

2 cups *Chinese Cabbage Ramen Salad* (see recipe on page 204) tossed with

3 oz. cooked chicken breast, chopped or shredded

AFTERNOON SNACK

½ cup *Yogurt Cucumber Sauce* (see recipe on page 324)

1 whole-wheat pita bread, toasted and cut into wedges

DINNER

1 serving *Crispy Baked Cod* (see recipe on page 217)

1 cup *Lentil Pilaf* (see recipe on page 258)

1 cup steamed broccoli

SNACK/DESSERT

½ cup *Maple Walnut Pudding* (see recipe on page 260)

1 oz. slivered almonds

If You're Not Breast-Feeding

REDUCE:

Peanut butter–filled pretzels to ½ oz. for Morning Snack

Lentil Pilaf to ½ cup for Dinner

ELIMINATE:

Slivered almonds for Snack/Dessert

MOVEMENT FOCUS

Today's **Movement Focus** is the Biceps Curl to strengthen your biceps. After all, you need strength to keep lifting that growing baby. While you're losing weight, your baby is growing! This is a new mom's variation on a traditional curl. It's most effective when done with a resistance band, but you can use an old bath towel until you get one.

Biceps Curl

❋ Sit in a chair for this biceps exercise.

❋ Place your foot on one end of the band or towel.

❋ Hold the other end in your fist and pull up, bending your elbow.

※ Hold for ten seconds and release. Keep your elbow close to the side of your body.

※ Do one set of five repetitions on each side.

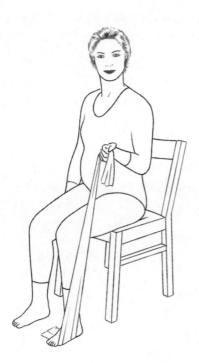

TODAY'S MOVEMENT PLAN

Kegels: as often as you can, at least twice a day

March in Place: three minutes

Shoulder Roll: ten repetitions, as often as you can

Neck Stretch: five repetitions, as often as you can

Reach and Crunch: five repetitions on each side

Waist Trimmer: five repetitions each side

Wall Push-ups: ten repetitions

Shoulder Blade Squeeze: ten repetitions on each side

Biceps Curl: five repetitions each arm, building to ten

Chest Stretch: three repetitions, anytime, but especially if your breasts feel heavy

March in Place: eight minutes

Leg Stretch: five repetitions with each leg

Day 16

Tonight's dinner will really spice things up! Studies show that the ground chile in the chili powder not only adds zest to a flavorful dish but also has wonderful benefits for the immune system, as red chiles are a good source of vitamins A and C. The *Chicken Fajitas* in today's dinner are a favorite for the former *Melrose Place* star and model Josie Bissett.

BREAKFAST

1 cup fat-free milk

1 cup fresh blackberries (if unavailable, substitute another berry with seeds)

1 slice *Cinnamon French Toast* (see recipe on page 210) with

2 Tbsp. wheat germ sprinkled on top

1 Tbsp. low-sugar maple syrup

MORNING SNACK

1 Tbsp. all-natural, reduced-fat peanut butter

6 whole-grain crackers

LUNCH

1 *Turkey Wrap* (see recipe on page 315)

1 apple or other seasonal fresh whole fruit

AFTERNOON SNACK

1 reduced-fat string cheese

2 cups air-popped popcorn

DINNER

1 serving *Chicken Fajitas* (see recipe on page 198)

1 whole-wheat tortilla

As much as you want of dark leafy greens as a salad with tomatoes, cucumbers, and your favorite veggies. (Make colorful choices for the most beneficial nutrients.)

1 Tbsp. low-fat (less than 5 g fat/serving) or fat-free salad dressing

SNACK/DESSERT

⅔ cup *Mexican Hot Cocoa* (see recipe on page 261)

If You're Not Breast-Feeding

REDUCE:

Peanut butter to 1½ tsp. for Morning Snack

Crackers to 3 for Morning Snack

Popcorn to 1 cup for Afternoon Snack

Chicken Fajitas to 4 oz. for Dinner

MOVEMENT FOCUS

Today's **Movement Focus** is an abdominal exercise that allows you to use the comfort of your bed: the Partial Sit-up.

Partial Sit-ups

✽ Lie on your back on the bed with your knees bent and your feet flat.

✽ With your hands behind your head, lift your elbows and upper body toward your knees and hold the movement at the top for a count of three.

✽ Slowly return to starting position.

✽ Do three sets of ten repetitions.

Remember since the bed sinks as you do each crunch, your abdominal muscles work harder to complete the move, so make sure you don't pull on your neck. Keep your elbows slightly forward, and your chin tucked in as you lift for the count of three.

TODAY'S MOVEMENT PLAN

Kegels: as often as you can, at least twice a day

March in Place: three minutes

Shoulder Roll: ten repetitions, as often as you can

Neck Stretch: five repetitions, as often as you can

Partial Sit-ups: three sets of ten repetitions

Waist Trimmer: five repetitions each side on each side

Wall Push-ups: ten repetitions

Shoulder Blade Squeeze: ten repetitions on each side

Biceps Curl: ten repetitions each arm

Chest Stretch: three repetitions, anytime, but especially if your breasts feel heavy

March in Place: eight minutes

Leg Stretch: five repetitions with each leg

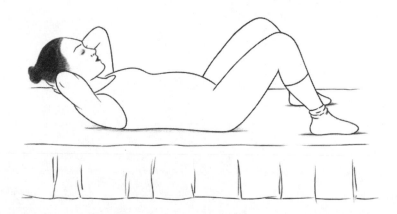

Day 17

Learning to manage portion sizes is key to maintaining a healthy weight. A 3-ounce portion of meat is the size of a deck of cards or the open palm of your hand (minus the fingers). A serving of vegetables is about the size of your fist. And a serving of pasta is about the size of one scoop of ice cream. A medium-size apple or other piece of fruit is about the size of a tennis ball. One serving of cheese is the size of a pair of dice or of a pink eraser. When it's not practical to accurately measure your portion size, you can "eyeball" it using the sizes that I've just described.

BREAKFAST

¾ cup bran flakes or equivalent cereal

1 cup fat-free milk

½ cup fresh blueberries, or 2 Tbsp. dried blueberries

MORNING SNACK

½ cup fat-free cottage cheese

3 prunes

LUNCH

1 serving *Eggplant Parmigiana* (see recipe on page 221)

1 large tomato, sliced

AFTERNOON SNACK

¼ cup pumpkin seeds

½ cup applesauce

DINNER

1 serving *Southwest Chicken and Veggie Salad* (see recipe on page 291) with

½ cup garbanzo beans on a bed of your choice of greens

1 whole-wheat flour tortilla

SNACK/DESSERT

2 store-bought gingersnaps

If You're Not Breast-Feeding

REDUCE:

Prunes to 2 for Morning Snack

Pumpkin seeds to 2 Tbsp. for Afternoon Snack

Southwest Chicken and Veggie Salad to 3 oz. for dinner

ELIMINATE:

Garbanzo beans at Dinner

MOVEMENT FOCUS

Are you remembering to do Kegels whenever you can? It's important to do them! Today's **Movement Focus** will add some inner thigh and buttocks strengthening to your workout with the Modified Pliés.

Modified Pliés

❋ Stand facing the back of a chair with your legs slightly wider than shoulder-width apart, toes pointed out to each side.

❋ Place both hands on the top of the back of the chair for support.

❋ Now, ballet style, keeping your back straight, bend your knees out to the side as far as you can comfortably while lowering your body toward the floor. Try to maintain constant tension in your legs as you perform this movement.

❋ Hold the position for ten seconds and then straighten your legs (without locking your knees), so you are back to the starting position.

❋ Repeat at least three times, more if you have the strength.

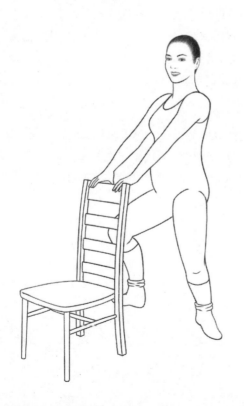

TODAY'S MOVEMENT PLAN

Kegels: as often as you can, at least twice a day

March in Place: three minutes

Shoulder Roll: ten repetitions, as often as you can

Neck Stretch: five repetitions, as often as you can

Partial Sit-ups: three sets of ten repetitions each

Waist Trimmer: five repetitions each side

Wall Push-ups: ten repetitions

Shoulder Blade Squeeze: ten repetitions on each side

Biceps Curl: ten repetitions each arm

Chest Stretch: three repetitions, anytime, but especially if your breasts feel heavy

Modified Pliés: at least three repetitions

March in Place: eight minutes

Leg Stretch: five repetitions with each leg

Day 18

Oatmeal is a great way to start the day. It is warm and delicious comfort food and gives you a wonderful morning energy boost! This is not the only great news; in addition, the FDA has approved the claim that "soluble fiber from oatmeal, as part of a low-saturated fat, low-cholesterol diet, may reduce the risk of heart disease."

Satisfying, gratifying *Pasta with Turkey Meat Sauce* is one of TV's Lauren Sanchez's favorites. Whether she's on Fox 11 News in Los Angeles or hosting the show *So You Think You Can Dance*, Lauren enjoys light, healthy food.

BREAKFAST

¾ cup calcium-fortified orange juice (or other calcium-fortified 100 percent fruit juice)

1 cup *Steel-Cut Oats* (see recipe on page 301) stirred with 2 Tbsp. wheat germ

4 Tbsp. raisins

1 cup fat-free milk

MORNING SNACK

1 slice whole-wheat toast

2 Tbsp. all-natural, reduced-fat peanut butter

LUNCH

1 serving *Fish with Sherry Mushroom Sauce* (see recipe on page 222)

½ ear corn on the cob

AFTERNOON SNACK

1 apple

½ oz. reduced-fat Monterey Jack cheese

DINNER

1½ cups *Pasta with Turkey Meat Sauce* (see recipe on page 268) (1 cup pasta and ½ cup meat sauce)

As much as you want of dark leafy greens as a salad with tomatoes, cucumbers, and your favorite veggies. (Make colorful choices for the most beneficial nutrients.)

1 Tbsp. low-fat (less than 5 g fat/serving) or fat-free salad dressing

SNACK/DESSERT

1 cup cut-up seasonal fruit

½ cup reduced-fat vanilla ice cream

If You're Not Breast-Feeding

REDUCE:

Raisins to 2 Tbsp. for Breakfast

Wheat germ to 1 Tbsp. for Breakfast

Peanut butter to 1½ tsp. for Morning Snack

Fish with Sherry Mushroom Sauce to 4 oz. for Lunch

MOVEMENT FOCUS

Our **Movement Focus** is the Hamstring Curl, which works the leg muscles.

Hamstring Curl

✽ Stand facing the back of a chair, with your hands holding the chair for balance.

✽ Bend your left knee and bring your right heel up as close to your buttocks as possible.

✽ Lower your foot to the ground and repeat. Do not lock your knee or release the contraction in your hamstring as you bend and straighten your leg.

✽ Repeat, using the right leg. Do three sets of fifteen repetitions with each leg.

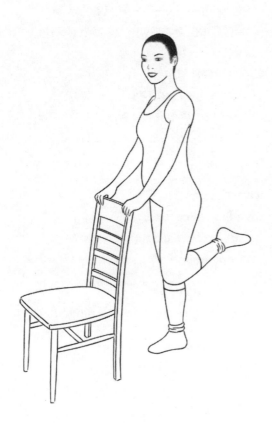

TODAY'S MOVEMENT PLAN

Kegels: as often as you can, at least twice a day

March in Place: three minutes

Shoulder Roll: ten repetitions, as often as you can

Neck Stretch: five repetitions, as often as you can

Partial Sit-ups: three sets of ten repetitions each

Waist Trimmer: five repetitions each side

Wall Push-ups: ten repetitions

Biceps Curl: ten repetitions each arm

Chest Stretch: three repetitions, anytime, but especially if your breasts feel heavy

Modified Pliés: at least three repetitions

Hamstring Curl: three sets of fifteen repetitions with each leg

March in Place: eight minutes

Leg Stretch: five repetitions with each leg

Day 19

Did you know that you have to eat seven cups of cornflakes to get the same amount of fiber as you get from eating one medium-sized orange? In addition to fiber, oranges are a great source of protein, calcium, iron, and vitamin C. That's why I've added an orange to this morning's breakfast menu. I've also included kiwi on today's menu because it's packed with even more vitamin C than an equivalent amount of orange.

Many a superstar loves the *Balsamic Broiled Salmon* on the menu tonight. It's appeared in the NutriFit menus of Uma Thurman, Angelina Jolie, Susan Sarandon, Charlize Theron, Marcia Gay Harden, and many others. Now, you'll be able to enjoy it, too.

BREAKFAST
1 *Bell Pepper and Cheese Omelet* (see recipe on page 188)
1 whole orange

MORNING SNACK
¼ cup *Cinnamon Spread* (see recipe on page 211) mixed with
1 Tbsp. wheat germ
6 whole-grain crackers

LUNCH
1 *Grilled Ham and Cheese Sandwich* (see recipe on page 241) on whole-wheat bread
1 cup fat-free milk

AFTERNOON SNACK
½ cup vanilla fat-free yogurt (or you may use plain)
1 kiwi

DINNER
1 serving *Balsamic Broiled Salmon* (see recipe on page 186)
½ cup *Brown Rice* (see recipe on page 196) sprinkled with
1 Tbsp. wheat germ
1 cup steamed cauliflower
1 cup *Spinach Salad with Honey Dijon Dressing* (see recipe on page 297)

SNACK/DESSERT
¾ cup *Chilled Apricot-Pear Soup* (see recipe on page 203)

If You're Not Breast-Feeding

REDUCE:
Bread to 1 slice for Lunch
Balsamic Broiled Salmon to 5 oz. for Dinner

SUBSTITUTE:
Carrots for crackers for Morning Snack

ELIMINATE:
Wheat germ at Dinner

MOVEMENT FOCUS

We are still focusing on the legs with today's **Movement Focus**, the Intensive Parallel Squat. It works your "saddle bags" area, the back of the legs and the buttocks.

Intensive Parallel Squat

❋ Stand with your legs shoulder-width apart and your back to the front of a chair.

❋ Keeping your back straight, slowly lower your buttocks toward the seat, as if you were planning to sit on its edge. Keep your stomach tight. When your butt touches the edge of the chair, straighten up slowly.

❋ Squeeze your buttocks just before you fully straighten your knees, making certain not to lock your joints and keeping the tension constant throughout the motion.

❋ Repeat five times or more if you can. Work up to twenty or thirty repetitions (but please, this one's tough, so only do as many as are comfortable in the beginning).

TODAY'S MOVEMENT PLAN

Kegels: as often as you can, at least twice a day

March in Place: three minutes

Shoulder Roll: ten repetitions, as often as you can

Neck Stretch: five repetitions, as often as you can

Partial Sit-ups: three sets of ten repetitions each

Waist Trimmer: five repetitions each side

Wall Push-ups: ten repetitions

Shoulder Blade Squeeze: ten repetitions on each side

Biceps Curl: ten repetitions each arm

Chest Stretch: three repetitions, anytime, but especially if your breasts feel heavy

Modified Pliés: at least three repetitions

Hamstring Curl: three sets of fifteen repetitions with each leg

Intensive Parallel Squat: at least five repetitions, building to twenty

March in Place: eight minutes

Leg Stretch: five repetitions with each leg

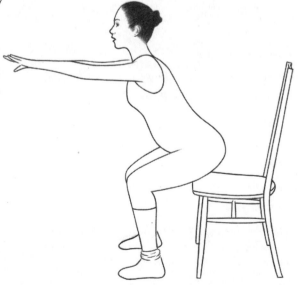

Day 20

There's delicious mashed yams on the dinner menu tonight. One cup of cubed, baked yam contains 24 percent of the daily value for vitamin B_6, an important vitamin for women. At least a dozen double-blind, placebo-controlled trials have demonstrated positive effects of vitamin B_6 in relieving PMS symptoms. Yams are a very good source of potassium, a mineral that helps to control blood pressure. Plus they taste delicious! Today is the last day of Phase 2 and if you'd like to see your progress, you can check your scale today—you'll have a pleasant surprise in store.

BREAKFAST

¾ cup whole-grain cold breakfast cereal (select one with at least 6 g dietary fiber and protein/serving)

½ cup blueberries

1 cup fat-free milk

MORNING SNACK

2 whole-grain rice cakes

1 Tbsp. all-natural, reduced-fat peanut butter

LUNCH

1 *Vegan Wrap* (see recipe on page 316)

½ cup strawberries

AFTERNOON SNACK

1 cup fat-free milk

2 whole-wheat fig bars

DINNER

1 serving *Aegean Cod* (see recipe on page 179)

1 cup *Chunky Mashed Yams* (see recipe on page 209)

½ cup *Grilled Vegetable Salad* (see recipe on page 244)

SNACK/DESSERT

1 cup sugar-free chocolate pudding

If You're Not Breast-Feeding

REDUCE:

Peanut butter to 1½ tsp. for Morning Snack

Fig bars to 1 fig bar for Afternoon Snack

Chunky Mashed Yams to ½ cup for Dinner

MOVEMENT FOCUS

Today's **Movement Focus** is the Backward Lunge, which will continue to strengthen your hamstrings and glutes.

Backward Lunge

❋ Open a door, and grasp the doorknobs on either side.

❋ Extend your left leg behind you, as if you are taking a long stride backward.

* Lift up onto the ball of your rear foot, shifting your weight onto the ball of that foot.

* Bend your left knee, squeeze your butt, and lower your body toward the ground to perform the lunge. Be sure that your weight is on the working leg, your right knee is directly over your right ankle, and your back knee is in line with your hip. Be careful not to hyperextend—that is, don't extend your front knee beyond the front toes. You needn't lunge very deeply at first to feel the workout in your hamstrings, glutes, and in the front of your thigh.

* Return to starting position and repeat with the right leg.

* Do one set of five repetitions with each leg, and work up to fifteen.

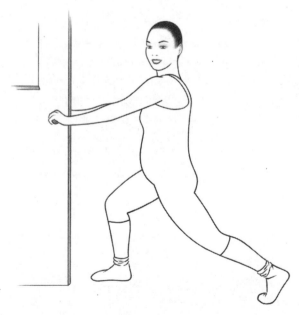

TODAY'S MOVEMENT PLAN

Kegels: as often as you can, at least twice a day

March in Place: three minutes

Shoulder Roll: ten repetitions, as often as you can

Neck Stretch: five repetitions, as often as you can

Partial Sit-ups: three sets of ten repetitions each

Waist Trimmer: five repetitions each side

Wall Push-ups: ten repetitions

Shoulder Blade Squeeze: ten repetitions on each side

Biceps Curl: ten repetitions each arm

Chest Stretch: three repetitions, anytime, but especially if your breasts feel heavy

Modified Pliés: at least three repetitions

Hamstring Curl: three sets of fifteen repetitions with each leg

Intensive Parallel Squat: at least five repetitions, building to twenty

Backward Lunge: five repetitions with each leg, building to fifteen

March in Place: eight minutes

Leg Stretch: five repetitions with each leg

h.a.l.t.s.

BEFORE moving on to Phase 3, let's revisit the **H.A.L.T.S.** system one last time, just to check in and see where you are.

Hungry? You may be feeling a little hungrier than normal. Try to zero in on where the hunger is coming from. Tune in to your emotions. Are you eating because you are bored? Instead of putting food in your mouth, now would be a great time to put the baby in a sling or the stroller and go for a few laps around the block. Maybe your body is sending you a signal that it's time for a quick snack. Don't feel guilty! Remember, in addition to your "mommy duties" you have been working out daily now for twenty consecutive days. Craving salt? Reach for a handful (about ten) of lower-sodium, whole-grain pretzels. Wish you could eat your favorite chocolate bar? A great guilt-free snack for these moments is fat-free chocolate pudding!

Angry? Give yourself a break. Make sure to set aside a few minutes each day to do something special just for you; after all, you can't always be Superwoman. Sneak a moment while the baby is down for a nap, put in your favorite soft CD, and make yourself a cup of chamomile tea; deep breathing exercises are also very helpful. Most important, know that it is just a feeling, we all experience it. And it, too, will pass!

Lonely? First, remind yourself that this is a perfectly normal feeling. Honor, acknowledge, and embrace it. The baby is now almost a month old; this would be a perfect time to look into joining a group for new mothers. You can find a group near you by looking in the phone book or online.

Tired? Don't you sometimes wish that you could sleep as much as your baby does? If you are feeling tired, take a moment to unwind. Relax in a hot bath or take a refreshing shower. As I mentioned, not being properly hydrated leads to fatigue. Have a tall glass of water. If you are getting tired of plain water, try one of the flavored waters on the market, or opt for a glass of sparkling water. Or reach for one of the high-water fruits like a handful of grapes, an orange, or an apple. You can make yourself a juice sparkler by mixing ½ cup of your favorite 100 percent fruit juice blend with ½ cup of plain club soda.

Stressed? Sometimes when we're stressed, the best thing we can do for ourselves is get playful. For a few moments, throw your cares away and play with your baby. Try doing some of the simple Mom and Baby movements in chapter 7. They're fun for you and for your baby. You need a break—and hearing your child laugh with you will help give you some perspective.

Day 21

Welcome to Day 1 of Phase 3. We're focusing on Super Performance. To ensure that you continue to increase your stamina, I'm adding the foods that contribute to increasing your strength. Look at what you've accomplished so far, in a very short time. And I know you're feeling good about your reflection in the mirror. Carbohydrates are a great source of fuel for the busy brain and body, so tonight pasta is on the menu! Actress Emmy Rossum of *Poseidon*, *The Day After Tomorrow,* and *The Phantom of the Opera* really loved this yummy *Linguine with Shrimp.*

BREAKFAST

½ cup coffee fat-free yogurt

1 slice whole-wheat bread, toasted

2 tsp. all-natural, reduced-fat peanut butter

½ cup cubed cantaloupe

MORNING SNACK

1 cup fat-free cottage cheese

1 cup pineapple, canned in juice, diced

LUNCH

1 *Grilled Chicken Breast Sandwich* (see recipe on page 239)

1 orange

AFTERNOON SNACK

1 reduced-fat string cheese

1 banana

DINNER

1 ¼ cups *Linguine with Shrimp* (see recipe on page 259)

As much as you want of dark leafy greens as a salad with tomatoes, cucumbers, and your favorite veggies. (Make colorful choices for the most beneficial nutrients.)

1 Tbsp. low-fat (less than 5 g fat/serving) or fat-free salad dressing

SNACK/DESSERT

2 *Raisin Oatmeal Cookies* (see recipe on page 281)

If You're Not Breast-Feeding

REDUCE:

Bread to 1 slice for Lunch

Banana to ½ for Afternoon Snack

Raisin Oatmeal Cookies to 1 cookie for Snack/Dessert

ELIMINATE:

Peanut butter at Breakfast

MOVEMENT FOCUS

Today's **Movement Focus** is the Standing Leg Lifts, which will build on yesterday's exercise by adding a new muscle to the regimen.

Standing Leg Lifts

❋ Stand next to a chair and hold on to it for balance.

❋ Keeping your body straight, lift your outer leg out to the side. As you lift up, keep your foot flexed and outer thigh muscle taut.

❋ Lower your leg, keeping your foot flexed and squeezing the inner thigh muscle as you bring the leg back to center.

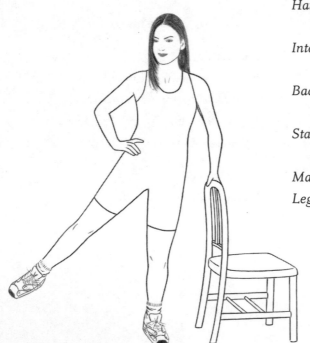

❋ Do one set of twenty repetitions. Now turn around and do one set of twenty repetitions with the other leg. If you can do another set, go for it!

TODAY'S MOVEMENT PLAN

Kegels: as often as you can, at least twice a day

March in Place: three minutes

Partial Sit-ups: three sets of ten repetitions each

Waist Trimmer: five repetitions each side

Wall Push-ups: ten repetitions

Biceps Curl: ten repetitions each arm

Chest Stretch: three repetitions, anytime, but especially if your breasts feel heavy

Modified Pliés: at least three repetitions

Hamstring Curl: three sets of fifteen repetitions with each leg

Intensive Parallel Squat: at least five repetitions, building to twenty

Backward Lunge: five repetitions with each leg, building to fifteen

Standing Leg Lifts: at least one set of twenty repetitions with each leg

March in Place: eight minutes

Leg Stretch: five repetitions with each leg

Day 22

Losing weight isn't always the goal of Nutri-Fit clients. A case in point is Penelope Cruz, who wanted healthy foods to play a more prominent role in her diet. She loved the Lemon-Grilled London Broil featured on today's menu, and it has also become a favorite of many *Body After Baby* moms.

A diet rich in fruits and vegetables has a plethora of benefits. If you are eating vegetables as one-third of your diet, you should notice that it is easier to achieve your body weight goals, as generous vegetable consumption helps fill the stomach faster, so you eat fewer high-calorie foods.

BREAKFAST

1 cup *Scrambled Eggs and Onions*
   (see recipe on page 288)
1 whole-wheat English muffin
1 tsp. trans fat–free light margarine or spread
1 cup fat-free milk

MORNING SNACK

1 apple
1 reduced-fat string cheese

LUNCH

1 veggie burger (store-bought) topped with
1 thin slice provolone, cheddar, or your
   favorite cheese on
1 sprouted whole-wheat bun with lettuce
   and tomatoes
1 cup cubed watermelon

AFTERNOON SNACK

½ cup *Yogurt Spread* (see recipe on page
   325) with
1 cup raw broccoli flowerets and
   cauliflowerets, or your favorite dippers

DINNER

1 serving *Lemon-Grilled London Broil*
   (see recipe on page 256)
1¼ cups *Roasted Vegetables* (see recipe on
   page 285)
1¼ cups *Spinach, Tomato, and Red-Onion
   Salad* (see recipe on page 300)

SNACK/DESSERT

12 animal crackers
1 cup fat-free milk

If You're Not Breast-Feeding

REDUCE:

English muffin to ½ for Breakfast
Burger bun to ½ for Lunch
Lemon-Grilled London Broil to 4 oz. for
   Dinner
Animal crackers to 6 for Snack/Dessert

MOVEMENT FOCUS

Today's **Movement Focus** is the Buttocks Lift, a great workout for your derriere.

Buttocks Lift

❀ Stand facing a wall and place your palms flat on the wall for balance.

❀ With your body straight and your stomach muscles tightened, extend your right leg out to the back, lifting your leg up as high as you can while keeping your foot flexed and your butt tight. Do not arch your back.

❀ Do one set of ten repetitions and work up to twenty. Repeat with the other leg. If you can do another set with each leg, do it!

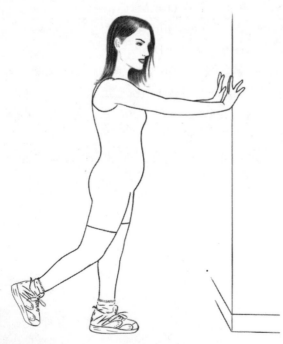

TODAY'S MOVEMENT PLAN

Kegels: as often as you can, at least twice a day

March in Place: three minutes

Partial Sit-ups: three sets of ten repetitions each

Waist Trimmer: five repetitions each side

Wall Push-ups: ten repetitions

Biceps Curl: ten repetitions each arm

Chest Stretch: three repetitions, anytime, but especially if your breasts feel heavy

Modified Pliés: at least three repetitions

Hamstring Curl: three sets of fifteen repetitions with each leg

Intensive Parallel Squat: at least five repetitions, building to twenty

Backward Lunge: five repetitions with each leg, building to fifteen

Standing Leg Lifts: at least twenty repetitions with each leg

Buttocks Lift: ten repetitions with each leg, building to twenty

March in Place: ten minutes

Leg Stretch: five repetitions with each leg

Day 23

Being weekend coanchor and correspondent for *Access Hollywood* keeps Shaun Robinson busy, so it's no wonder that she enjoyed having NutriFit prepare many of her meals, including the *Pork Chops with Onions and Apples*. By now you probably understand that the recipes you're eating on my plan are the same nutritious meals that many of my clients and their families eat all the time. They're simple to prepare, so you'll not only enjoy eating them, you'll also enjoy making them!

BREAKFAST

1 cup rolled oats, cooked according to package directions, mixed with
2 Tbsp. wheat germ and topped with
1 cup fresh berries (whatever is in season)
1 cup fat-free milk

MORNING SNACK

½ grapefruit
2 Tbsp. Neufchâtel light cream cheese
6 whole-grain crackers

LUNCH

1 *Open-faced Turkey Club Sandwich* (see recipe on page 263)
1 cup fat-free milk

AFTERNOON SNACK

1 cup instant miso soup (look for a lower-sodium package)

DINNER

1 serving *Pork Chops with Onions and Apples* (see recipe on page 277)
1 cup sautéed green beans
1 tomato, sliced and topped with a splash of balsamic vinegar
½ cup wild rice

SNACK/DESSERT

1 cup *Chocolate Tofu Pudding* (see recipe on page 208)

If You're Not Breast-Feeding

REDUCE:

Wheat germ to 1 Tbsp. for Breakfast
Cream cheese to 1 Tbsp. for Morning Snack
Crackers to 3 for Morning Snack
Pork Chops with Onions and Apples to 4 oz. for Dinner
Chocolate Tofu Pudding to ½ cup for Snack/Dessert

MOVEMENT FOCUS

Today's **Movement Focus** is the Standing Waist Squeeze, which helps trim your waist.

Standing Waist Squeeze

❋ Stand with your legs slightly more than shoulder-width apart, toes turned out slightly. Keep your knees slightly bent.

❋ Place your left arm behind your head and bend your upper body sideways to the right. Hold the stretch for the count of three and return to the starting position.

❋ Do one set of ten reaches on each side.

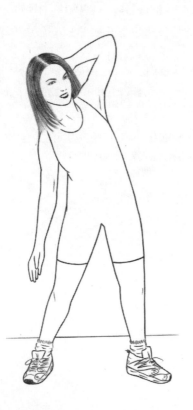

TODAY'S MOVEMENT PLAN

Kegels: as often as you can, at least twice a day

March in Place: three minutes

Partial Sit-ups: three sets of ten repetitions each

Waist Trimmer: five repetitions each side

Wall Push-ups: ten repetitions

Biceps Curl: ten repetitions each arm

Chest Stretch: three repetitions, anytime, but especially if your breasts feel heavy

Modified Pliés: at least three repetitions

Hamstring Curl: three sets of fifteen repetitions with each leg

Backward Lunge: five repetitions with each leg, building to fifteen

Standing Leg Lifts: at least twenty repetitions with each leg

Standing Waist Squeeze: ten repetitions each side

March in Place: ten minutes

Leg Stretch: five repetitions with each leg

Day 24

Shamicka Lawrence (Mrs. Martin Lawrence) always keeps her energy level on high with a good breakfast. The *Fresh Spinach Omelet* that you'll have today is one of her favorites. Spinach gives you a lot of the iron you need to get through these busy days.

I personally love the *Roasted Tomato Soup*, which is so easy, flavorful, and low in calories! The recipe makes 6 servings, so freeze the leftovers in 1-cup containers and enjoy it again on Days 26 and 30. I'll bet that this will be one of your favorite recipes.

BREAKFAST

1 cup prune juice, ¼ cup prunes, or 1 Tbsp. blackstrap molasses
1 *Fresh Spinach Omelet* (see recipe on page 229)
1 slice whole-wheat bread, toasted
1 kiwi

MORNING SNACK

½ cup fat-free cottage cheese
1 cup strawberries

LUNCH

1 ¼ cups *Roasted Tomato Soup* (see recipe on page 284)
1 whole-wheat roll and 1 oz. reduced-fat cheddar cheese
As much as you want of dark leafy greens as a salad with tomatoes, cucumbers, and your favorite veggies. (Make colorful choices for the most beneficial nutrients. Top with 2 Tbsp. wheat germ.)
1 Tbsp. low-fat (less than 5 g fat/serving) or fat-free salad dressing

AFTERNOON SNACK

1 cup fat-free milk
1 Asian pear

DINNER

1 serving *Baja-Style Cod with Salsa Coulis* (see recipe on page 184)
1 cup brown rice
½ cup steamed vegetables (your choice)

SNACK/DESSERT

2 slices *Warm Pineapple Rings* (see recipe on page 321)

If You're Not Breast-Feeding

REDUCE:

Whole-wheat roll to ½ for Lunch
Baja-Style Cod with Salsa Coulis to 5 oz. fish for Dinner
Brown rice to ½ cup for Dinner

ELIMINATE:

Wheat germ at Lunch

MOVEMENT FOCUS

Today's **Movement Focus** is the Hip Thrust, which will continue to work your gluteus and hamstring muscles.

Hip Thrusts

❋ Lie on your back and bend your knees, placing your feet flat on the floor, shoulder-width apart.

❋ Relax your upper back and head, and slowly lift your hips up off the floor, squeezing your buttocks as you lift.

❋ Hold for the count of ten, supporting your weight on your shoulder blades, then lower gently back to the floor, one vertebra at a time.

❋ Repeat. Work up to two sets of ten repetitions.

TODAY'S MOVEMENT PLAN

Kegels: as often as you can, at least twice a day

March in Place: three minutes

Partial Sit-ups: three sets of ten repetitions each

Waist Trimmer: five repetitions each side

Hip Thrust: ten repetitions, building to two sets of ten repetitions

Wall Push-ups: ten repetitions

Biceps Curl: ten repetitions each arm

Chest Stretch: three repetitions, anytime, but especially if your breasts feel heavy

Modified Pliés: at least three repetitions

Hamstring Curl: three sets of fifteen repetitions with each leg

Buttocks Lift: ten repetitions with each leg, building to twenty

Backward Lunge: five repetitions with each leg, building to fifteen

Standing Leg Lifts: at least twenty repetitions with each leg

Standing Waist Squeeze: ten repetitions each side

March in Place: ten minutes

Leg Stretch: five repetitions with each leg

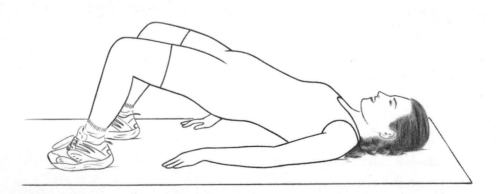

Day 25

A fresh grapefruit is an amazing midmorning snack. Grapefruits are low in calories, low in sodium, high in potassium, and high in fat-burning enzymes. Another positive benefit of eating grapefruit is the high water content. Grapefruits are almost 90 percent water. Eating any fruit with a high water content helps boost your hydration level, and increasing water consumption also makes it easier for your digestive tract to work properly.

And the savory *Ginger Garlic Tofu* on today's menu is rich in phytochemicals that not only enhance your body's natural healing process, but provide complete proteins.

BREAKFAST

1 serving whole-grain frozen waffles

1 Tbsp. light maple syrup

½ cup raspberries

1 cup fat-free milk

MORNING SNACK

2 tsp. all-natural, reduced-fat peanut butter

1 whole-grain rice cake

½ grapefruit

LUNCH

4 oz. *Ginger Garlic Tofu* (see recipe on page 234)

¼ cup rice noodles

1 ¼ cups *Black Bean Salad* (see recipe on page 189)

AFTERNOON SNACK

1 oz. walnuts

½ cup vanilla fat-free yogurt

DINNER

1 serving *Grilled Chicken Breast* (see recipe on page 238)

½ cup *Fragrant Brown Rice and Peas* (see recipe on page 223)

1 cup fat-free milk

SNACK/DESSERT

½ cup *Strawberries Italiano* (see recipe on page 302)

If You're Not Breast-Feeding

REDUCE:

Black Bean Salad to ½ cup for Lunch

Walnuts to ½ oz. for Afternoon Snack

Grilled Chicken Breast to 4 oz. for Dinner

MOVEMENT FOCUS

Today's **Movement Focus** is the Upright Row, which strengthens your front and shoulder muscles (deltoids) and upper back. You can perform this exercise holding light weights (2 lbs.), soup cans, or filled small plastic water bottles.

Upright Row

✤ Standing up, start by holding the weights in front of your thighs (your knuckles should be pointing forward).

✤ Now bring your hands to your chest as shown in the illustration; your upper arms will be parallel to the floor if you're doing this rowing motion properly.

✤ Return slowly to the starting position.

✤ Do one set of ten repetitions.

TODAY'S MOVEMENT PLAN

Kegels: as often as you can, at least twice a day

March in Place: three minutes

Partial Sit-ups: three sets of ten repetitions each

Waist Trimmer: five repetitions each side

Hip Thrust: ten repetitions, building to two sets of ten repetitions

Wall Push-ups: ten repetitions

Biceps Curl: ten repetitions each arm

Upright Row: ten repetitions

Chest Stretch: three repetitions, anytime, but especially if your breasts feel heavy

Modified Pliés: at least three repetitions

Hamstring Curl: three sets of fifteen repetitions with each leg

Buttocks Lift: ten repetitions with each leg, building to twenty

Backward Lunge: five repetitions with each leg, building to fifteen

Standing Leg Lifts: at least twenty repetitions with each leg

Standing Waist Squeeze: ten repetitions each side

March in Place: ten minutes

Leg Stretch: five repetitions with each leg

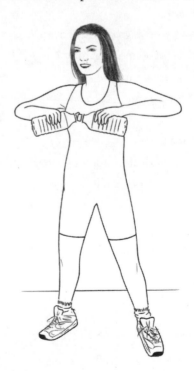

Day 26

Tonight's menu features trout for dinner because trout is rich in omega-3 fatty acids, which have a whole range of health benefits, including protection against heart disease, stroke, arthritis, and psoriasis. Recent studies show that breast-feeding women should eat between one and two portions of oily fish a week, and should do so not just for the health benefits but because oily fish also helps the neurological development of their babies!

BREAKFAST

1 cup *Swedish Muesli* (see recipe on
    page 305)
½ cup macadamia nuts

MORNING SNACK

1 pear
1 oz. reduced-fat string cheese

LUNCH

1 ¼ cups *Roasted Tomato Soup* (defrost a
    frozen portion you prepared on Day 24)
1 *Grilled Turkey Breast Sandwich* (see
    recipe on page 243)

AFTERNOON SNACK

1 oz. roasted almonds

DINNER

1 serving *Fresh Baked Rainbow Trout*
    (see recipe on page 226), sautéed with
1 Tbsp. toasted pine nuts
½ cup baked yam
⅔ cup *Zucchini with Mushrooms* (see
    recipe on page 326)

SNACK/DESSERT

1 cup *Peach and Berry Crisp* (see recipe on
    page 271)

If You're Not Breast-Feeding

REDUCE:

Bread to 1 slice for Lunch

ELIMINATE:

Macadamia nuts at Breakfast
Pine nuts at Dinner

MOVEMENT FOCUS

Today's **Movement Focus** is the Triceps Extension, which will work and define the triceps.

Triceps Extension

❀ Stand with your left knee bent, resting on the seat of a chair.

❀ Bend forward at the waist and support yourself by holding the back of the chair with your right hand.

❀ Keeping your left elbow close to your side and your fist loosely clenched, lift your elbow up and extend your forearm and hand back and up toward the ceiling.

❋ Return to starting position.

❋ Do ten repetitions. Reverse the position and perform ten repetitions with the other arm.

TODAY'S MOVEMENT PLAN

Kegels: as often as you can, at least twice a day

March in Place: three minutes

Partial Sit-ups: three sets of ten repetitions each

Hip Thrust: ten repetitions, building to two sets of ten repetitions

Wall Push-ups: ten repetitions

Biceps Curl: ten repetitions each arm

Tricep Extension: ten repetitions with each arm

Upright Row: ten repetitions

Chest Stretch: three repetitions, anytime, but especially if your breasts feel heavy

Modified Pliés: at least three repetitions

Hamstring Curl: three sets of fifteen repetitions with each leg

Buttocks Lift: ten repetitions with each leg, building to twenty

Backward Lunge: five repetitions with each leg, building to fifteen

Standing Leg Lifts: at least twenty repetitions with each leg

Standing Waist Squeeze: ten repetitions each side

March in Place: twelve minutes

Leg Stretch: five repetitions with each leg

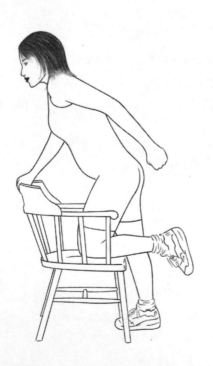

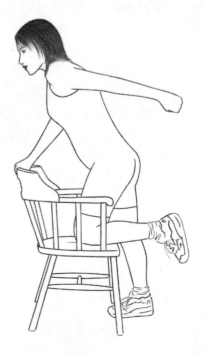

Day 27

You'll notice that today, like many days, we've started the day with whole-grain cereal, a food rich in dietary fiber. Not only is whole-grain cereal a great source of energy for a new mom, but it also plays a key role in maintaining the health of your digestive system. Foods rich in dietary fiber also help you feel full faster and longer. Dietary fiber allows your body to absorb carbohydrates more slowly, helping to keep blood sugar levels stable and energy constant.

Academy Award–winner Marcia Gay Harden wanted to get back to her prepregnancy weight when she started with Nutri-Fit meals. I provided her with dishes like the *Baked Turkey Dijon* to help her regain her beautiful figure. Marcia was one of my inspirations for the *Body After Baby* plan.

BREAKFAST
1 cup whole-grain breakfast cereal
    (use one with at least 6 g dietary fiber
    and protein/serving)
½ whole banana
1 cup fat-free milk

MORNING SNACK
2 Tbsp. all-natural, reduced-fat
    peanut butter
4 celery sticks
4 Tbsp. raisins

LUNCH
2 servings *Greek Egg Scramble* (see recipe
    on page 235)
6 whole-grain crackers

AFTERNOON SNACK
1 cup vanilla fat-free yogurt
1 cup fresh berries

DINNER
1 serving *Baked Turkey Dijon* (see recipe
    on page 185)
1 cup *Asparagus Broccoli Bouquet*
    (see recipe on page 183)
½ baked potato with skin
As much as you want of dark leafy greens
    as a salad with tomatoes, cucumbers,
    and your favorite veggies. (Make color-
    ful choices for the most beneficial nu-
    trients.)
1 Tbsp. low-fat (less than 5 g fat/serving)
    or fat-free salad dressing

SNACK/DESSERT
1 cup fat-free milk
6 reduced-fat vanilla wafers

If You're Not Breast-Feeding

REDUCE:

Peanut butter to 1 Tbsp. for Morning Snack

Raisins to 1 Tbsp. for Morning Snack

Baked Turkey Dijon to 3 oz. for Dinner

Baked potato to ¼ potato for Dinner

Vanilla wafers to 3 for Snack/Dessert

MOVEMENT FOCUS

Today's **Movement Focus** is the Single Leg Crunch, which will tighten both the upper and lower abdominal muscles.

Single Leg Crunch

❋ Lying on your back on the floor, extend one leg straight up in the air; bend the other leg so that your foot is flat on the ground.

❋ Clasp your hands behind your head, elbows forward, and support your head without pulling on your neck.

❋ Gently lift your shoulders off the floor, tightening your abs as you lift your chest toward your leg, keeping your chin tucked in.

❋ Do fifteen repetitions, then switch legs and repeat.

❋ Work up to two sets of fifteen repetitions on each side.

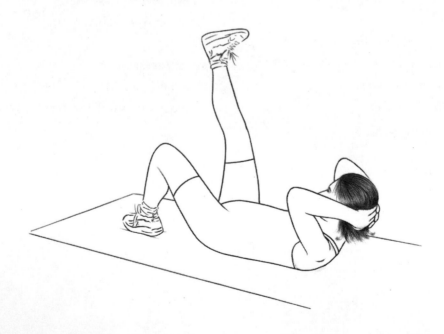

TODAY'S MOVEMENT PLAN

Kegels: as often as you can, at least twice a day

March in Place: three minutes

Partial Sit-ups: three sets of ten repetitions each

Single Leg Crunch: fifteen repetitions on each side, building to two sets of fifteen repetitions

Hip Thrust: ten repetitions, building to two sets of ten repetitions

Wall Push-ups: ten repetitions

Shoulder Blade Squeeze: ten repetitions

Biceps Curl: ten repetitions each arm

Triceps Extension: ten repetitions with each arm

Upright Row: ten repetitions

Chest Stretch: three repetitions, anytime, but especially if your breasts feel heavy

Modified Pliés: at least three repetitions

Hamstring Curl: three sets of fifteen repetitions with each leg

Buttocks Lift: ten repetitions with each leg, building to twenty

Backward Lunge: five repetitions with each leg, building to fifteen

Standing Leg Lifts: at least twenty repetitions with each leg

Standing Waist Squeeze: ten repetitions each side

March in Place: twelve minutes

Leg Stretch: five repetitions with each leg

Day 28

Today it's time to go to the market again, but this time, look back over the various meals you've enjoyed for the last few weeks and develop your own shopping list. In two days, you'll be designing your own plan, so you can shop for it now. I'm sure there were certain dishes that you put on your "WOW-gotta-have-that-again!" list; put those ingredients on your list so you'll be prepared. Have fun!

BREAKFAST

1 serving (2 eggs) *Huevos Rancheros*
    (see recipe on page 250)
2 corn tortillas, slightly warmed
¾ cup calcium-fortified orange juice
    (or other 100 percent fruit, calcium-fortified juice)

MORNING SNACK

1 *Turkey Burger* patty (see recipe on page 313) with
1 sliced tomato
1 dill pickle

LUNCH

1 serving *Garbanzo Pita Pockets* (see recipe on page 233)
1 peach
1 cup fat-free milk

AFTERNOON SNACK

½ cup strawberry frozen yogurt topped with 2 tsp. Grape-Nuts cereal

DINNER

1 serving *Thai Basil Chicken* (see recipe on page 307)
1 cup steamed snow peas
½ cup brown rice

SNACK/DESSERT

2 *Oatmeal Chocolate Chip Cookies* (see recipe on page 262)

If You're Not Breast-Feeding

REDUCE:

Huevos Rancheros to 1 egg for Breakfast
Corn tortillas to 1 tortilla for Breakfast
Thai Basil Chicken to 3 oz. for Dinner
Oatmeal Chocolate Chip Cookies to 1 cookie for Snack/Dessert

SUBSTITUTE:

½ cup fat-free cottage cheese for *Turkey Burger*

MOVEMENT FOCUS

Today's **Movement Focus** is the Wall Squat, an isometric exercise that uses the wall for support.

Wall Squat

❋ Lean with your back against the wall and walk your feet out about 18 inches in front of the wall. You can let your arms hang loosely by your side or fold them across your chest.

❋ Slide your body down the wall into a squat; your thighs should be parallel to the floor.

❋ Do three reps; hold each for ten seconds, then slide up to the starting position. Work up to holding the position for twenty seconds. If you can hold the movement longer, you'll get even more benefit from it.

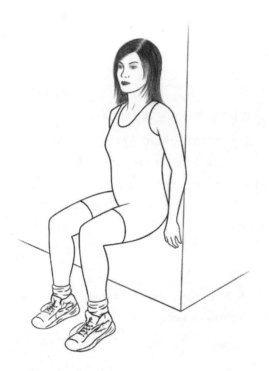

TODAY'S MOVEMENT PLAN

Kegels: as often as you can, at least twice a day

March in Place: three minutes

Partial Sit-ups: three sets of ten repetitions each

Single Leg Crunch: fifteen repetitions each side, building to two sets of fifteen repetitions

Wall Push-ups: ten repetitions

Biceps Curl: ten repetitions each arm

Triceps Extension: ten repetitions with each arm

Upright Row: ten repetitions

Chest Stretch: three repetitions, anytime, but especially if your breasts feel heavy

Modified Pliés: at least three repetitions

Buttocks Lift: ten repetitions with each leg, building to twenty

Backward Lunge: five repetitions with each leg, building to fifteen

Standing Leg Lifts: at least twenty repetitions with each leg

Wall Squat: three repetitions of ten seconds each, building to twenty seconds

Standing Waist Squeeze: ten repetitions each side

March in Place: twelve minutes

Leg Stretch: five repetitions with each leg

Day 29

Can you believe that this is already Day 29! You are nurturing your child and yourself, and you're determined and focused. Congratulations.

BREAKFAST

½ cup *Fruit-and-Nut Granola* (see recipe on page 232) mixed with

2 Tbsp. wheat germ

1 cup fat-free milk

1 banana

MORNING SNACK

1 reduced-fat string cheese

1 kiwi

LUNCH

1 serving *Greek Pita Pizza* (see recipe on page 237)

1¼ cups *Spinach, Tomato, and Red-Onion Salad* (see recipe on page 300)

AFTERNOON SNACK

1 pear

1 oz. whole-grain pretzels

DINNER

1 serving *Rockin' Moroccan Sirloin Roast* (see recipe on page 286)

1 small steamed red potato

1 cup *Fragrant Kale* (see recipe on page 224)

1 cup fat-free milk

SNACK/DESSERT

1 *Spiced Baked Apple with Walnuts* (see recipe on page 293)

If You're Not Breast-Feeding

REDUCE:

Wheat germ to 1 Tbsp. for Breakfast

Banana to ½ for Breakfast

Rockin' Moroccan Sirloin Roast to 4 oz. for Dinner

ELIMINATE:

Pretzels at Afternoon Snack

MOVEMENT FOCUS

Today's **Movement Focus** is the Neck Press, which helps strengthen the muscles in your neck. You'll need a folded hand towel to do this exercise. The Neck Press is a great way to finish each day's workout.

Neck Press

❋ Stand about arm's distance from a wall, or slightly closer.

❋ Lean forward, bringing your forehead to the wall and use the towel to cushion your forehead. Your body should be at approximately a 45-degree angle. Do not use your hands for support (you can clasp them loosely behind your back or let them hang at your sides).

❋ Hold for thirty seconds, then work up to one minute.

❃ Now, turn around and lean the back of your head against the towel and walk your feet out in front of you as far as you can. You'll feel some tension in your neck as you perform this movement; it's strengthening your neck with every second that you hold the position.

❃ When you have finished one set (front and back), stand up very straight and tall against the wall with your heels and shoulders right up to the wall.

❃ Press your shoulders back against the wall.

❃ Tuck your buttocks and hold for thirty seconds.

❃ Keeping your chin level, walk forward ten feet and feel how your posture has improved. Walk lightly as though you are floating on air.

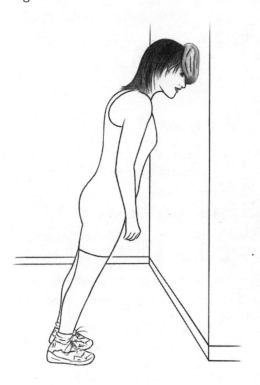

TODAY'S MOVEMENT PLAN

Kegels: as often as you can, at least twice a day

March in Place: three minutes

Partial Sit-ups: three sets of ten repetitions each

Single Leg Crunch: fifteen repetitions, building to two sets of fifteen repetitions

Wall Push-ups: ten repetitions

Biceps Curl: ten repetitions each arm

Triceps Extension: ten repetitions with each arm

Upright Row: ten repetitions

Chest Stretch: three repetitions, anytime, but especially if your breasts feel heavy

Modified Pliés: at least three repetitions

Buttocks Lift: ten repetitions with each leg, building to twenty

Backward Lunge: five repetitions with each leg, building to fifteen

Standing Leg Lifts: at least twenty repetitions with each leg

Wall Squat: three repetitions of ten seconds each, building to twenty seconds

Standing Waist Squeeze: ten repetitions each side

March in Place: twelve minutes

Leg Stretch: five repetitions with each leg

Neck Press: thirty seconds each position

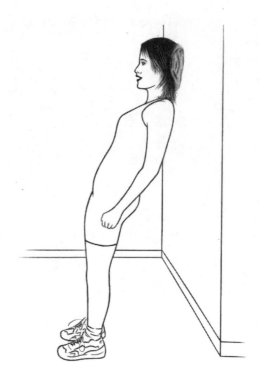

Day 30

You did it! Today is the last day of your *Body After Baby* plan. You've learned good eating habits and you've had remarkable success. Check the scale. Measure your success! If you still have more weight to drop, you know how to do it. Now you can create your own menu plans or repeat the *Body After Baby* plan until you reach your weight-loss goal. However, now that you're closer to your goal (and many of you have reached your goal), your rate of weight loss will be slower. But it's a safe plan to use over and over again, starting at Day 1 and working through to Day 30. This morning celebrate the last day of the plan with a delicious bowl of fresh fruit and cottage cheese, sprinkled with a few almonds.

BREAKFAST

1 cup *Fresh Seasonal Fruit Salad* (see recipe on page 228) with
1 cup fat-free cottage cheese and
2 Tbsp. slivered almonds
½ whole-wheat English muffin, toasted
1 Tbsp. 100 percent all-fruit preserves

MORNING SNACK

1 orange
½ cup fat-free yogurt

LUNCH

¾ cup *Chicken Salad with Spiced Sesame Sauce* (see recipe on page 200) on a bed of as much as you want of dark leafy greens as a salad with tomatoes, cucumbers, and your favorite veggies. (Make colorful choices for the most beneficial nutrients.)
1 Tbsp. low-fat (less than 5 g fat/serving) or fat-free salad dressing
1 ¼ cups *Roasted Tomato Soup* (defrost a frozen portion you prepared on Day 24)

AFTERNOON SNACK

1 cup cubed honeydew melon

DINNER

2 cups *Spinach, Tofu, and Brown Rice Stir-fry* (see recipe on page 299)
1 cup beets (roasted)

SNACK/DESSERT

1 slice *Chocolate Pecan Cake* (see recipe on page 207)
1 cup fat-free milk

If You're Not Breast-Feeding

REDUCE:
Roasted Tomato Soup to 1 cup for Lunch
Spinach, Tofu, and Brown Rice Stir-fry to 1 cup for Dinner
Chocolate Pecan Cake to ½ slice for Snack/Dessert

MOVEMENT FOCUS

Today's **Movement Focus** is the Spin-Around Jump, which may be the most challenging one yet! You'll need supportive shoes, so grab those tennies.

Spin-Around Jump

❀ Start in a standing position. Jump up while turning around 180 degrees so you land on both feet, facing in the opposite direction.

❀ Reverse the movement and jump back around to your starting position.

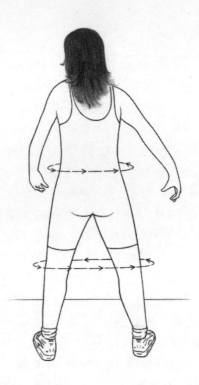

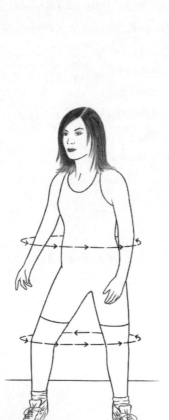

❀ Repeat the exercise, turning to the opposite side.

❀ Do ten turns to each side, alternating sides with each jump. Try to land lightly on your feet, keeping your knees slightly bent for proper shock absorption.

Below is the **Movement Plan** you can now do every day to stay fit and to continue sculpting your body.

This **Movement Plan** contains something for each major muscle group and can help you sustain and strengthen your new body. As you continue to grow stronger and become more active, you can add light weights, resistance bands, and other ergonomic aids to provide a more challenging workout. This will allow for progression and increased resistance, two essential elements that must be present for continued strengthening. Vary the exercises and add additional cardio/aerobic activities to your routine to prevent getting bored. Have fun and enjoy your renewed Body After Baby!

THE MOVEMENT PLAN

Kegels: as often as you can, at least twice a day

March in Place (Day 10): three minute warm-up, then two 12–14-minute intervals whenever you can

Partial Sit-ups (Day 16): two sets, twenty repetitions each

Single Leg Crunches (Day 27): two sets, fifteen repetitions each leg

Wall Push-ups (Day 13): two sets, twenty repetitions each

Biceps Curl (Day 15): two sets (with band), ten repetitions each arm

Triceps Extension (Day 26): two sets, ten repetitions each arm

Upright Row (Day 25): two sets, ten repetitions each arm

Chest Stretch (Day 6): twice a day, thirty seconds at a time

Modified Pliés (Day 17): two sets, fifteen repetitions each

Buttocks Lift (Day 22): two sets, fifteen repetitions each

Backward Lunge (Day 20): two sets, fifteen repetitions each

Standing Waist Squeeze (Day 23): two sets, fifteen repetitions each side

Neck Stretch (Day 8): twice a day, thirty seconds at a time

Shoulder Rolls (Day 7): at least twice a day, ten repetitions each; anytime you need a stress relief

Spin-Around Jumps (Day 30): two sets, ten times each

Leg Stretch (Day 9): after you complete the exercises

Neck Press (Day 29): two sets, one minute each segment

alternative *body after* *baby* plans

FOR YOU VEGETARIAN MOMS, this 15-day plan provides all of the important complete proteins that you'll need to stay strong and healthy. After the first two weeks, repeat the plan. Follow the same exercise plan as in the regular *Body After Baby* plan. For those of you who are just home from the hospital with your new baby, you may be feeling a bit overwhelmed. That's how many moms feel—even if this isn't your first child, or second, or third. . . . Take heart, the abbreviated Jumpstart plan on page 138 will really help you get your energy back and prepare you to tackle the full 30-day plan when you are ready.

THE 15-DAY VEGETARIAN PLAN

You can definitely be a vegetarian or vegan and adhere to the *Body After Baby* plan when you are breast-feeding. Just be aware of a few things suggested by La Leche League, the breast-feeding specialists:

- If your diet contains no animal protein whatsoever, increase your soy intake and whole-grain cereals fortified with B_{12}. You also may want to speak to your doctor about vitamin B$_{12}$ supplements. If the baby is deficient in this important B vitamin, you may observe a loss of appetite, lethargy, vomiting, or weakness. Discuss this immediately with your health-care professional.

- If you do not drink milk or dairy products, eat as many other calcium-rich foods as possible. You'll find that certain foods, such as ¼ cup of ground sesame seeds, have as much calcium as a glass of milk. And many greens are very rich in this important nutrient. You can also up your calcium intake with blackstrap molasses, soy products, dark leafy greens, and nuts, such as almonds and Brazil nuts. To increase your vitamin D levels, take more walks in the sun and look for vitamin D–enriched foods such as whole-grain cereals and juices.

Day 1

BREAKFAST
1 cup calcium-fortified orange juice
 (or other 100 percent fruit, calcium-
 fortified juice)
1 poached egg (or you can have it prepared
 any other way, without additional fat)
1 slice whole-wheat bread, toasted
1 tsp. trans fat–free light margarine or
 spread
½ cup blueberries

MORNING SNACK
½ large apple, sliced
¼ cup pumpkin seeds

LUNCH
4 oz. *Ginger Garlic Tofu* (see recipe on
 page 234)
½ cup brown rice

AFTERNOON SNACK
1 cup *Black Bean Salad* (see recipe
 on page 189)

DINNER
1 cup *Sweet Potato Curry with Lentils*
 (see recipe on page 306)
½ cup steamed Swiss chard

SNACK/DESSERT
3 Tbsp. *Chocolate Chip Fondue* (see recipe
 on page 205)
2 graham crackers

If You're Not Breast-Feeding

REDUCE:
Pumpkin seeds to 2 Tbsp. at Morning
 Snack
Black Bean Salad to ½ cup at Afternoon
 Snack
Graham crackers to 1 at Snack/Dessert

Day 2

BREAKFAST

1 cup whole-grain breakfast cereal (use one
with at least 6 g dietary fiber and
protein/serving)

1 cup fat-free milk

¼ whole banana, sliced

½ cup blueberries

MORNING SNACK

1 orange

½ oz. pistachio nuts

LUNCH

1 serving *Garbanzo Pita Pockets* (see recipe
on page 233)

2 cups *Spinach Salad with Honey Dijon
Dressing* (see recipe on page 297)

AFTERNOON SNACK

½ cup *Power Snack Mix* (see recipe on
page 279)

DINNER

2½ cups *Peanut Noodles and Veggies*
(see recipe on page 275)

1 cup *Asian Cucumber Salad* (see recipe on
page 182)

SNACK/DESSERT

12 animal crackers

1 cup fat-free milk

If You're Not Breast-Feeding

REDUCE:

Power Snack Mix to ¼ cup at Afternoon
Snack

Peanut Noodles and Veggies to 1½ cups at
Dinner

Animal crackers to 6 at Snack/Dessert

Day 3

BREAKFAST

1 cup calcium-fortified orange juice
(or other 100 percent fruit, calcium-
fortified juice)

½ cup instant oatmeal, prepared according
to package directions, substituting

½ cup unsweetened apple juice for water

½ cup chopped fresh apple, stirred into
oatmeal for sweetening

1 cup fat-free milk

MORNING SNACK

4 Tbsp. dried fruit, such as raisins

1 oz. almonds

LUNCH

1 cup *Quinoa Super Salad* (see recipe on
page 280) on a bed of as much as you
want of dark leafy greens as a salad
with tomatoes, cucumbers, and your
favorite veggies. (Make colorful choices
for the most beneficial nutrients.)

1 Tbsp. low-fat (less than 5 g fat/serving)
or fat-free salad dressing

AFTERNOON SNACK

1 pear

1 oz. peanuts

DINNER

1 serving *Fresh Tomato Salad* (see recipe on
page 230) sprinkled with

1 tsp. pine nuts

2 cups *Stuffed Squash with Cheese*
(see recipe on page 304)

1 cup steamed broccoli

SNACK/DESSERT

½ cup reduced-fat chocolate ice cream

½ cup sliced fresh strawberries

If You're Not Breast-Feeding

REDUCE:

Almonds to ½ oz. at Morning Snack

Peanuts to ½ oz. at Afternoon Snack

Stuffed Squash with Cheese to 1½ cups at
Dinner

Chocolate ice cream to ¼ cup at
Snack/Dessert

Day 4

BREAKFAST
1 *Bran Raisin Muffin* (see recipe on page 195, or use small store-bought variety, made with whole grains)
2 egg whites, scrambled with
1 whole egg
1 cup fat-free milk

MORNING SNACK
½ cup grapes
2 celery sticks
2 Tbsp. Neufchâtel light cream cheese

LUNCH
1 serving (2) *Vegetarian Bean Enchiladas* (see recipe on page 319) mixed with
2 Tbsp. wheat germ
1 cup sliced zucchini

AFTERNOON SNACK
1 Asian pear
1 oz. peanuts

DINNER
2 servings *Stuffed Portobello Mushrooms* (see recipe on page 303)
1 cup *Fragrant Kale* (see recipe on page 224)

SNACK/DESSERT
½ cup vanilla fat-free yogurt
½ cup blueberries

If You're Not Breast-Feeding

REDUCE:
Neufchâtel cream cheese to 1 Tbsp. at Morning Snack
Wheat germ to 1 Tbsp. at Lunch
Peanuts to ½ oz. at Afternoon Snack
Fat-free yogurt to ¼ cup at Snack/Dessert

Day 5

BREAKFAST

1 cup calcium-fortified orange juice
(or other 100 percent fruit,
calcium-fortified juice)

1 *Peanut Butter and Jelly Sandwich*
(see recipe on page 272)

MORNING SNACK

½ cup fat-free cottage cheese

1 cup juice-packed fruit cocktail, or 1 cup
cut-up fresh fruit salad

1 Tbsp. chopped walnuts

LUNCH

2 cups *Ratatouille* (see recipe
on page 282)

½ cup brown rice

AFTERNOON SNACK

1 apple

1 reduced-fat string cheese

DINNER

1½ cups *Kale and Millet Stew* (see recipe
on page 252)

1 cup green beans

As much as you want of dark leafy greens
as a salad with tomatoes, cucumbers,
and your favorite veggies. (Make colorful choices for the most beneficial
nutrients.)

2 Tbsp. low-fat (less than 5 g fat/serving)
or fat-free salad dressing

SNACK/DESSERT

1 oz. whole-grain pretzels

2 Tbsp. semisweet chocolate chips

If You're Not Breast-Feeding

REDUCE:

Brown rice to ¼ cup at Lunch

Pretzels to ½ oz. at Snack/Dessert

Chocolate chips to 1 Tbsp. at
Snack/Dessert

ELIMINATE:

Walnuts at Morning Snack

Day 6

BREAKFAST

1 serving (2 slices) *High-Protein French Toast* (see recipe on page 247)

½ grapefruit

1 cup fat-free milk

MORNING SNACK

½ cup fat-free cottage cheese

2 cups cubed cantaloupe and honeydew melons

LUNCH

1 cup *Black-eyed Pea and Legume Salad* (see recipe on page 192) with

2 Tbsp. wheat germ mixed in

1 cup *Spinach, Tomato, and Red-Onion Salad* (see recipe on page 300)

AFTERNOON SNACK

2 oz. roasted soy nuts

DINNER

Pasta with Vegetarian Meatballs (see recipe on page 269) with ½ cup pasta and ½ cup marinara sauce (store-bought)

1 cup steamed green beans

SNACK/DESSERT

¼ cup *Piña Colada Dip* (see recipe on page 276)

1 banana

If You're Not Breast-Feeding

REDUCE:

Wheat germ to 1 Tbsp. at Lunch

Soy nuts to 1 oz. at Afternoon Snack

Day 7

BREAKFAST

1 *Cheese Omelet* (see recipe on page 197)

½ whole-wheat English muffin

1 tsp. 100 percent all-fruit preserves

1 orange

MORNING SNACK

One 4-inch serving *Lavosh Wrap with Hummus and Veggies* (see recipe on page 254)

1 apple

LUNCH

2 cups *Black Bean, Corn, and Barley Salad* (see recipe on page 191) on 2 cups assorted greens

AFTERNOON SNACK

½ cup peanut butter–filled pretzels

1 cup fat-free milk

DINNER

2 servings *Eggplant Parmigiana* (see recipe on page 221)

1 cup steamed summer squash

1 cup *Tomato, Mozzarella, and Basil Salad* (see recipe on page 311)

SNACK/DESSERT

One 3-inch slice *Angel Food Cake* (see recipe on page 180)

½ cup sliced fresh strawberries

If You're Not Breast-Feeding

REDUCE:

Black Bean, Corn, and Barley Salad to 1 cup for Lunch

Peanut butter pretzels to ¼ cup for Afternoon Snack

Eggplant Parmigiana to 1 serving for Dinner

ELIMINATE:

Apple at Morning Snack

Day 8

BREAKFAST

1 cup prune juice, or 1 Tbsp. blackstrap
 molasses
½ cup *Couscous with Raisins and Dates*
 (see recipe on page 215)
1 cup fat-free milk

MORNING SNACK

1 cup fruit-flavored fat-free yogurt

LUNCH

1 cup *Fried Rice with Soybeans* (see recipe
 on page 231)
1 cup cut-up fresh fruit salad

AFTERNOON SNACK

¼ cup *Herb Dip* (see recipe on page 245)
1 cup raw veggies for dipping, your choice

DINNER

1 cup *Vegetable Barley Soup* (see recipe on
 page 317)
8 pieces store-bought vegetarian "chicken"
 nuggets
½ baked potato
1 cup steamed spinach

SNACK/DESSERT

½ cup vanilla fat-free frozen yogurt

If You're Not Breast-Feeding

REDUCE:
Yogurt to ½ cup for Morning Snack
Vegetable Barley Soup to ½ cup for Dinner
Vegetarian "chicken" nuggets to 6 pieces
 for Dinner

Day 9

BREAKFAST

¾ cup whole-grain cold cereal (use one
   with at least 6 g dietary fiber and pro-
   tein/serving), topped with

½ cup blueberries

1 cup fat-free milk

MORNING SNACK

5 oz. *Wild Berry Smoothie* (see recipe on
   page 322) blended with

2 Tbsp. wheat germ

LUNCH

1½ servings *Lasagna Roll-ups* (see recipe
   on page 253)

As much as you want of dark leafy greens
   as a salad with tomatoes, cucumbers,
   and your favorite veggies. (Make colorful choices for the most beneficial nutrients.)

1 Tbsp. low-fat (less than 5 g fat/serving)
   or fat-free salad dressing

AFTERNOON SNACK

2 oz. almonds

DINNER

1¼ cups *Spinach, Tomato, and Red-Onion
   Salad* (see recipe on page 300) with
   1 Tbsp. low-fat (less than 5 g fat/serving)
   or fat-free salad dressing

1½ cups *Pasta with Black Beans* (see
   recipe on page 266)

1 cup cooked carrots

SNACK/DESSERT

1 store-bought biscotti

1 cup fat-free milk

If You're Not Breast-Feeding

REDUCE:

Wheat germ to 1 Tbsp. for Morning Snack

Lasagna Roll-ups to 1 serving for Lunch

Almonds to 1 oz. for Afternoon Snack

Pasta with Black Beans to 1 cup for Dinner

Day 10

BREAKFAST

¾ cup calcium-fortified orange juice
(or other 100 percent fruit, calcium-
fortified juice)

1 banana

1 small whole-wheat bagel

2 oz. fat-free cream cheese

½ grapefruit

MORNING SNACK

1 cup *Greek Feta Salad* (see recipe on
page 236)

LUNCH

2 servings *Spinach, Cheese, and Mushroom Bake* (see recipe on page 298)

2 cups fresh fruit (at least 1 cup strawberries, plus 1 cup fruit of your choice)

AFTERNOON SNACK

1 serving *Egg Salad* (see recipe on
page 219)

6 whole-grain crackers

DINNER

1 serving *Couscous-Stuffed Squash*
(see recipe on page 214)

½ cup mushrooms sautéed in

2 tsp. extra-virgin olive oil

As much as you want of dark leafy greens
as a salad with tomatoes, cucumbers,
and your favorite veggies. (Make colorful choices for the most beneficial
nutrients.)

Sprinkle with 2 Tbsp. wheat germ

2 Tbsp. *Creamy Herb Dressing* (see recipe
on page 216)

SNACK/DESSERT

2 Tbsp. *Peanut Butter–Hot Fudge Dip*
(see recipe on page 273)

2 squares low-fat graham crackers

If You're Not Breast-Feeding

REDUCE:

Spinach, Cheese, and Mushroom Bake
to 1 serving for Lunch

Whole-grain crackers to 3 for Afternoon
Snack

Wheat germ to 1 Tbsp. for Dinner

Peanut Butter–Hot Fudge Dip to 1 Tbsp.
for Snack/Dessert

Graham crackers to 1 square for
Snack/Dessert

Day 11

BREAKFAST

1 orange

One 3-inch square *Blueberry Lemon Coffee Cake* (see recipe on page 193)

1 cup fat-free milk

MORNING SNACK

1 medium peach

1 cup fruit-flavored fat-free yogurt

LUNCH

1½ cups *Pasta with White Beans* (see recipe on page 270)

As much as you want of dark leafy greens as a salad with tomatoes, cucumbers, and your favorite veggies. (Make colorful choices for the most beneficial nutrients.)

1 Tbsp. low-fat (less than 5 g fat/serving) or fat-free salad dressing

AFTERNOON SNACK

¼ cup *Artichoke Dip* (see recipe on page 181)

1 cup baby carrots

DINNER

1 cup *Asian Cucumber Salad* (see recipe on page 182)

1 cup *Tofu Hoisin with Vegetables and Walnuts* (see recipe on page 309)

1 cup cooked spinach

SNACK/DESSERT

1 serving store-bought, sugar-free chocolate pudding

If You're Not Breast-Feeding

REDUCE:

Blueberry Lemon Coffee Cake to 2-inch square

Yogurt to ½ cup at Morning Snack

Pasta with White Beans to ½ cup for Lunch

Day 12

BREAKFAST

1 cup prune juice

4 *Blueberry Whole-Wheat Pancakes*
(see recipe on page 194)

2 scrambled egg whites

1 cup fat-free milk

MORNING SNACK

½ cup fruit-flavored fat-free yogurt

1 apple, sliced

LUNCH

1 cup *Eggless Egg Salad* (see recipe on page
220), as a sandwich on

2 slices whole-wheat bread with

1 tomato, sliced, and

1 cup lettuce leaves

AFTERNOON SNACK

¼ cup *Black Bean Salad* (see recipe on
page 189)

1 cup jicama sticks

DINNER

1 cup *Fragrant Lentil Soup* (see recipe on
page 225) (freeze leftovers in 1-cup
container for Day 14)

1½ cups *Tomato, Potato, and Eggplant
Gratin* (see recipe on page 312)

1 cup steamed broccoli

SNACK/DESSERT

2-inch square *Chocolate Chip Spice Cake*
(see recipe on page 206)

If You're Not Breast-Feeding

REDUCE:

Blueberry Whole-Wheat Pancakes
to 2 for Breakfast

Whole-wheat bread to 1 slice at Lunch

Tomato, Potato, and Eggplant Gratin
to 1 cup for Dinner

Chocolate Chip Spice Cake to 1½-inch
square for Snack/Dessert

Day 13

BREAKFAST

1 cup cubed cantaloupe melon, sprinkled
  with 2 Tbsp. wheat germ
1 whole-wheat bagel
1 Tbsp. all-natural, reduced-fat
  peanut butter

MORNING SNACK

½ cup grapes
1 cup fat-free milk

LUNCH

1 serving *Vegetarian Enchilada Casserole*
  (see recipe on page 320)
As much as you want of dark leafy greens
  as a salad with tomatoes, cucumbers,
  and your favorite veggies. (Make colorful choices for the most beneficial nutrients.)
1 Tbsp. low-fat (less than 5 g fat/serving)
  or fat-free salad dressing

AFTERNOON SNACK

¼ cup *Spinach and Chive Dip* (see recipe
  on page 295)
1 cup jicama sticks

DINNER

1¼ cups *Roasted Tomato Soup* (see recipe
  on page 284)
1½ cups *Fresh Herb Risotto with Peas*
  (see recipe on page 227)
1 cup steamed green beans

SNACK/DESSERT

½ cup fat-free frozen yogurt, your favorite
  flavor
1 nectarine

If You're Not Breast-Feeding

REDUCE:

Wheat germ to 1 Tbsp. for Breakfast
Bagel to ½ for Breakfast
Fresh Herb Risotto with Peas to 1 cup for
  Dinner

Day 14

BREAKFAST
1 Tbsp. blackstrap molasses
1 *Spanish Omelet* (see recipe on page 292)
1 small whole-wheat tortilla
1 orange

MORNING SNACK
1½ oz. *Holiday Cheese Log* (see recipe on page 248)
1 apple, cut into wedges

LUNCH
1½ cups *Fragrant Lentil Soup* (defrost a frozen portion you prepared on Day 12)
6 whole-grain crackers
1 cup raw veggies, your favorite

AFTERNOON SNACK
2 *Cocoa Fruit Nougats* (see recipe on page 212)
1 cup fat-free milk

DINNER
1½ cups *Spinach, Tofu, and Brown Rice Stir-fry* (see recipe on page 299)
1 cup steamed cauliflower
As much as you want of dark leafy greens as a salad with tomatoes, cucumbers, and your favorite veggies. (Make colorful choices for the most beneficial nutrients.)
1 Tbsp. low-fat (less than 5 g fat/serving) or fat-free salad dressing

SNACK/DESSERT
6 wedges *Dessert Nachos* (see recipe on page 218)

If You're Not Breast-Feeding

REDUCE:
Fragrant Lentil Soup to 1 cup for Lunch
Crackers to 3 for Lunch
Cocoa Fruit Nuggets to 1 for Afternoon Snack
Dessert Nachos to 3 wedges for Snack/Dessert

Day 15

BREAKFAST

1 cup *Banana and Orange Oatmeal*
(see recipe on page 187)
1 Tbsp. wheat germ (stir into oatmeal)
1 cup fat-free milk

MORNING SNACK

1 oz. whole-grain pretzels

LUNCH

1 cup *Tofu Chili* (see recipe on page 308)
1 Tbsp. wheat germ (stir into chili)
1 cup steamed green beans

AFTERNOON SNACK

½ cup *Yogurt Cucumber Sauce* (see recipe
on page 324)
1 whole-wheat pita bread, cut into quarters
and toasted

DINNER

1 cup *Pasta with Dilled Pea Sauce*
(see recipe on page 267)
1 cup steamed broccoli
1½ cups *Spinach, Tomato, and Red-Onion
Salad* (see recipe on page 300)

SNACK/DESSERT

½ cup *Maple Walnut Pudding* (see recipe
on page 260)
2 Tbsp. slivered almonds

If You're Not Breast-Feeding

REDUCE:

Pretzels to ½ oz. for Morning Snack
Maple Walnut Pudding to ¼ cup for
Snack/Dessert
Almonds to 1 Tbsp. for Snack/Dessert

ELIMINATE:

Wheat germ at Breakfast

The 10-Day Jumpstart Plan

If you don't have time to think about your grocery shopping and trying new recipes, I understand your situation and have created this chapter for you. Remember, your hormones are sending signals to your body that it's time to lose weight. In order to take advantage of such a receptive internal environment, I've designed a 10-day Jumpstart meal plan that you can begin right now. You probably have all the food right now in your pantry or refrigerator. It's a complete, healthy plan—with 1,800-2,000 nutrient-dense calories per day—so nursing (and non-nursing) mothers will be well fed. And, of course, it's absolutely simple. If you're not nursing, just skip the morning snack. You won't be hungry, and you'll be energized, even-keeled, and ready to handle anything!

You can repeat this 10-day plan as often as you wish, but if you're like me, you'll probably start to crave variety before very long. I'm sure you'll want to know how the right foods will help you heal, and why the *Body After Baby* plan works. In chapters 2 and 3, I explain all those things and more—especially, why it's important to eat certain foods to help with the specific health concerns of new moms. These foods will help you sleep better, provide you with plenty of energy, and actually help you shed pounds faster. When you're ready, advance to my 30-day plan. Get ready for results—the *Body After Baby* way!

Right now, though, enjoy these ten days of quick-and-easy, no-think meals—menus that will restore your energy and satisfy your appetite so you can stay focused on your beautiful new child!

Day 1

BREAKFAST

1 slice whole-wheat toast

1 egg, scrambled in a nonstick skillet sprayed with cooking spray

1 cup fresh berries

1 cup nonfat milk

MORNING SNACK

1 banana

8 oz. nonfat vanilla yogurt

10 almonds

1 cup green tea

LUNCH

Grilled Chicken Salad

2 oz. grilled skinless and boneless chicken, sliced

2 cups salad greens, tomatoes, cucumbers, radishes, carrots (or your favorite colorful veggies)

1 Tbsp. low-fat (less than 5 g fat/serving) dressing

1 slice whole-grain bread, cut into cubes and toasted

1 Tbsp. shredded Parmesan cheese

1 orange

AFTERNOON SNACK

1 corn tortilla filled with:

½ cup canned kidney beans, rinsed and drained

1 oz. low-fat cheddar cheese, shredded

2 Tbsp. salsa

DINNER

Chinese Stir-Fry with Shrimp

1½ cups frozen or fresh ready-to-cook stir-fry vegetables, sautéed in

2 tsp. canola oil with

3 oz. ready-to-cook shrimp, seasoned with dash of reduced-sodium soy sauce

½ cup cooked whole-grain soba noodles or ½ cup cooked brown rice

EVENING SNACK

Baked Apple

1 apple filled with:

1 Tbsp. chopped walnuts and raisins, mixed with dash of cinnamon

Bake at 350°F for 20 minutes, or until soft

1 cup green tea

Day 2

BREAKFAST
1 cup whole-grain breakfast cereal
½ cup blueberries
½ cup sliced strawberries
1 cup nonfat milk (for the cereal)

MORNING SNACK
1 can sliced pineapple, unsweetened, juice-
   packed
1 cup nonfat cottage cheese
1 cup green tea

LUNCH
Veggie Wrap
1 whole-wheat flour tortilla
2 oz. low-fat cheese
½ cup cooked black beans
1 cup bell peppers, sliced and cooked
⅓ fresh avocado
½ cup torn fresh spinach leaves
¼ cup fresh tomato salsa

handful of baby carrots
1 cup green tea

AFTERNOON SNACK
1 slice whole-wheat bread topped with:
1 Tbsp. peanut butter
1 banana, sliced

DINNER
5 oz. orange roughy, red snapper, or sole,
   pan-sautéed with 1 tsp. olive oil, seasoned with salt, pepper, and lemon juice
1 cup pan-grilled bell peppers and zucchini,
   or your favorite green vegetables
2 cups salad greens, tomatoes, cucumbers,
   radishes, carrots (or your favorite
   colorful veggies)
1 Tbsp. low-fat (less than 5 g fat/serving)
   dressing
½ cup baked yam
1 cup nonfat milk

EVENING SNACK
¾ cup low-fat frozen yogurt
1 cup green tea

Day 3

BREAKFAST

1 cup cooked oatmeal, with 1 tsp. brown
    sugar and ½ cup nonfat milk
1 cup berries
1 cup orange juice

MORNING SNACK

1 rice cake topped with 1 Tbsp. reduced-fat,
    all-natural peanut butter
1 banana
1 cup fresh cherries or other fruit

LUNCH

Barley Pilaf

½ cup pearl barley, cooked according to
    package directions
1 cup vegetables (fresh spinach leaves,
    diced red bell peppers, chopped onions)
    sautéed with:
3 oz. low-fat turkey sausage, thinly sliced
    into rounds, mixed into the barley

1 cup reduced-sodium V8 juice

AFTERNOON SNACK

1 fresh pear
10 almonds or cashews
1 cup green tea

DINNER

1½ cups cooked linguine topped with:
3 oz. grilled scallops
2 cups chopped and lightly steamed
    vegetables, tossed with 1 Tbsp. olive oil
2 Tbsp. grated Parmesan cheese

2 cups salad greens, tomatoes, cucumbers,
    radishes, carrots (or your favorite
    colorful veggies)
1 Tbsp. low-fat (less than 5 g fat/serving)
    dressing

1 cup green tea

EVENING SNACK

1 cup fat-free chocolate pudding
    (store-bought)

Day 4

BREAKFAST

Cheese Omelet

1 cup fat-free egg substitute

1 oz. low-fat cheddar or Monterey Jack cheese

Cook in a nonstick skillet sprayed with cooking spray.

2 slices whole-grain toast

1 cup orange juice

MORNING SNACK

1 cup sliced strawberries

1 kiwi, peeled (or unpeeled) and sliced

6 oz. nonfat yogurt

LUNCH

1½ cups lentil soup, store-bought (Select one with less than 350 mg sodium/serving.)

½ whole-wheat roll or 4 whole-wheat crackers

1 apple

1 cup nonfat milk

AFTERNOON SNACK

1 pear

10 walnut halves

1 cup green tea

DINNER

4 oz. salmon, broiled with lemon and dill

½ cup brown rice

1 cup steamed vegetables

1 cup sliced peppers/jicama/carrots, mixed with 1 Tbsp. low-fat dressing

EVENING SNACK

1 cup sugar-free hot cocoa (packaged mix), made with 1 cup nonfat milk

Day 5

BREAKFAST

Fresh Fruit and Cottage Cheese

½ cup fresh papaya or mango

½ cup honeydew or watermelon chunks

½ cup cantaloupe chunks

½ cup fresh grapes or strawberries

1 cup nonfat cottage cheese

10 almonds

1 slice raisin toast, spread with 1 tsp. all-fruit jam

MORNING SNACK

Lavosh Wrap with Peanut Butter/Tofu Filling

1 serving of fresh whole-wheat lavosh or 1 whole-wheat tortilla, spread with:

2 Tbsp. filling made by mixing equal parts peanut butter with reduced-fat tofu (Refrigerate unused filling for later treat.)

Top with:

½ banana, thinly sliced, or 1 Tbsp. dried mixed-fruit bits

LUNCH

Turkey Sandwich

3 oz. smoked turkey breast

1 tsp. mustard, mixed with 1 tsp. fat-free mayonnaise

1 lettuce leaf

2 slices whole-grain bread

½ cup three-bean salad (or use canned variety)

1 cup nonfat milk

AFTERNOON SNACK

6 whole-wheat crackers

1 oz. reduced-fat cheese

DINNER

3 oz. grilled chicken breast

2 cups salad greens, tomatoes, cucumbers, radishes, carrots (or your favorite colorful veggies)

1 Tbsp. low-fat (less than 5 g fat/serving) dressing

½ cup cooked rice (wild, brown, or your favorite medley of whole-grain rice)

1 cup nonfat milk

EVENING SNACK

Peach Crisp

1 cup sliced peaches (with skin), topped with:

2 Tbsp. quick oats, mixed with:

1 Tbsp. frozen pineapple or apple-juice concentrate (undiluted)

Dash cinnamon

Sprinkle topping over peach slices and bake at 350°F for 15 minutes, or until bubbling.

1 cup green tea

Day 6

BREAKFAST

2 eggs, scrambled (in a nonstick pan
    sprayed with cooking spray) with:

¼ cup diced bell pepper

¼ cup chopped tomato

¼ cup chopped mushroom

1 oz. reduced-fat cheese

¼ whole-wheat bagel, spread with:

1 tsp. trans fat–free light margarine or
    fat-free cream cheese

1 cup green tea

MORNING SNACK

Piña Colada Dip

½ cup vanilla yogurt mixed with:

2 Tbsp. unsweetened, crushed pineapple, in
    juice (You may add a drop of coconut
    extract.)

1 tsp. honey

1 banana, cut into chunks or thin slices, for
    dipping

LUNCH

Grilled Chicken Caesar Salad

3 oz. grilled chicken breast

2 cups romaine lettuce

¼ cup toasted whole-wheat croutons

1 oz. shredded Parmesan cheese

2 Tbsp. low-fat Caesar dressing

1 cup mixed cherry tomatoes and red
    bell pepper strips

1 tangerine

AFTERNOON SNACK

1 cup fat-free yogurt

1 oz. (2 Tbsp.) roasted soy nuts

5 dried apricot halves

1 cup green tea

DINNER

Shrimp Fajitas

3 oz. fresh, medium-sized shrimp, cooked

1 tomato, cut into chunks

1 cup fresh bell pepper strips

¼ cup thinly sliced mushrooms

Sauté in 1 tsp. olive oil; add chili powder
    and hot pepper sauce.

2 corn tortillas

1 cup nonfat milk

EVENING SNACK

½ cup vanilla frozen yogurt

½ cup raspberries

Day 7

BREAKFAST

1 whole-wheat English muffin

2 tsp. trans fat–free light margarine or
fat-free cream cheese

2 hard-boiled eggs

1 cup fresh grapes

1 cup nonfat milk

MORNING SNACK

4 bread sticks

1 oz. string cheese

LUNCH

Legume Vegetable Salad

1 cup canned legumes (such as beans,
lentils, or green peas)

1 cup vegetables (such as carrots, celery,
and bell peppers), diced

1 Tbsp. minced red onion

1 Tbsp. Italian parsley, chopped

1 Tbsp. balsamic vinegar

1 Tbsp. olive oil

1 cup nonfat milk

2 oatmeal raisin cookies

AFTERNOON SNACK

2 cups watermelon cubes

DINNER

4 oz. lean pork chop baked with:

1 Tbsp. barbecue sauce (350°F for 15
minutes, or until done)

1 small baked potato, topped with:

1 Tbsp. nonfat sour cream or
1 tsp. trans fat–free light margarine

1 cup fresh baby carrots and summer
squash, steamed

2 cups salad greens, tomatoes, cucumbers,
radishes, carrots (or your favorite colorful veggies) tossed with:

1 Tbsp. low-fat (less than 5 g fat/serving)
dressing

EVENING SNACK

1 cup low-fat tapioca pudding
(store-bought)

1 cup green tea

Day 8

BREAKFAST

1 slice (¾ oz.) provolone, Swiss, or cheddar
   cheese
1 whole-wheat bagel with 1 tsp. trans
   fat–free light margarine
½ cup grapefruit juice

MORNING SNACK

½ cup plain yogurt
1 apple

LUNCH

Salmon Pocket
1 whole-wheat pita bread (8 in.), filled with:
2 oz. canned salmon
¼ cup chopped cucumber
1 tsp. fat-free mayonnaise
lemon juice, black pepper to taste

½ cup nonfat milk

AFTERNOON SNACK

1 pear
1 oz. string cheese

DINNER

3 oz. roast beef
½ cup mashed potatoes (with 1 tsp. trans
   fat–free margarine, 2 Tbsp. nonfat
   milk)
½ cup cooked broccoli
½ cup cooked cauliflower
2 cups salad greens, tomatoes, cucumbers,
   radishes, carrots (or your favorite colorful veggies), tossed with:
1 Tbsp. low-fat (less than 5 g fat/serving)
   dressing

EVENING SNACK

1 orange
1 oz. roasted soy nuts

Day 9

BREAKFAST

¾ cup whole-grain cereal

1 cup nonfat milk

½ banana, sliced

1 tsp. slivered almonds

MORNING SNACK

6 whole-grain crackers

1 hard-boiled egg

1 cup green tea

LUNCH

Turkey Club Sandwich

2 oz. roast turkey

1 slice turkey bacon, halved

¼ avocado, thinly sliced

½ tomato, thinly sliced

2 pieces lettuce, rinsed and patted dry

2 slices whole-wheat bread, spread with:

1 tsp. fat-free mayonnaise

½ cup raw baby carrots

AFTERNOON SNACK

1 cup nonfat yogurt

½ cup berries

DINNER

3 oz. grilled lamb chop

½ cup baked yams

½ cup green beans

2 cups salad greens, tomatoes, cucumbers, radishes, and carrots (or your favorite colorful veggies), tossed with:

1 Tbsp. low-fat (less than 5 g fat/serving) dressing

EVENING SNACK

¼ cup trail mix

1 cup green tea

Day 10

BREAKFAST
2 frozen whole-grain waffles (store-bought)
1 Tbsp. reduced-sugar pancake syrup
½ cup sliced berries
2 reduced-fat turkey breakfast sausages
½ cup calcium-fortified orange juice

MORNING SNACK
1 plum, nectarine or peach
1 oz. almonds
1 cup green tea

LUNCH
Grilled Cheese Sandwich
2 slices 2 percent American cheese
2 slices whole-wheat bread
1 tsp. trans fat–free margarine

1 cup grapes
1 cup nonfat milk

AFTERNOON SNACK
3 cups air-popped popcorn (or reduced-fat, store-bought popcorn)

DINNER
4 oz. grilled salmon, cod, or trout
½ cup cooked brown rice
1 cup steamed spinach
2 cups green salad, topped with:
Shredded red cabbage, carrots, and cherry tomatoes, tossed with:
1 Tbsp. oil-and-vinegar-style dressing

1 cup nonfat milk

EVENING SNACK
½ cup reduced-fat ice cream or 1 oz. dark chocolate
1 cup green tea

jumpstart meal plan tips

RELAX! This meal plan is intended to make healthy eating as simple as can be. Here are ten easy tips that will help you plan and shop for this phase of your *Body After Baby* success.

1. If you don't like fish, substitute chicken or turkey. Fish has wonderful healthy fats, however, so you may want to consider adding an omega-3 fatty acid supplement to your prenatal vitamins, which you should still be taking (per your physician's recommendation). You can do the same if you substitute beef, lamb, and pork in the meal plan.

2. If you don't like milk as a beverage, consider trying reduced-fat soymilk as a substitute. Remember, dairy products are a good source of calcium, so try to incorporate yogurt and cheese in your meal plan to ensure adequate amounts of calcium in your diet.

3. Think "color" when you choose your fruits and vegetables. Go for the darkest greens, the deepest blues and purples, the most vivacious reds and oranges, the brightest yellows—these fruits and vegetables will generally have a higher vitamin and mineral content. Add variety and, if there's something in the plan that's out of season or unavailable, feel free to substitute another fruit or vegetable.

4. Choose whole-grain breads and cereals and experiment with bran, brown rice, rye, pumpernickel, or the newest addition to the whole-grain family, white whole wheat. Select a variety that has the most fiber per slice or serving.

5. When purchasing salad dressings, choose lower-fat options, and oil and vinegar–based dressings. Those made with olive oil will be among the healthiest choices you can make.

6. Steaming vegetables is super simple! You can steam using a microwave oven by putting a tiny amount of water in a glass or microwave-safe bowl, and covering it with paper towels or microwave-safe plastic wrap.

7. All of these meal plans are designed for one serving. If you'd like to add more servings for your children or partner, simply multiply the quantities as many times as you need. You may want to adjust the protein portion size for anyone who's not trying to lose a little weight or for growing children.

8. Green tea is included daily for its favorable phytonutrients and disease-protective properties. You can select decaffeinated green tea if you prefer, but "regular" green tea is fine, too, as are the flavored varieties. Try to drink at least two cups every day.

9. You may drink coffee in moderation (up to two cups daily), but try to avoid alcoholic beverages. Make sure you drink plenty of water (at least eight glasses daily).

10. If you're hungry, add a piece of fruit or some raw vegetables. If you're going out to dinner or are invited to a party, have a piece of fruit before you go and make the best selections you can at the event. Try to stick close to the meal plan.

common questions about
the *body after baby* plan

HERE ARE THE ANSWERS to questions that *Body After Baby* clients frequently ask about the plan:

Q | *Is it safe to be dieting right after delivery?*
A | "Dieting" in a highly restrictive way is rarely appropriate, and especially not a good idea if you're a postpartum mom. The *Body After Baby* plan is not a restrictive diet; it's a nutritionally balanced eating program that provides all the essential nutrients that the mother of a newborn needs, and it's safe. This regimen is a well-rounded, healthy way to eat for the rest of your life, and you can begin the day you get home from the hospital. The plan includes a balance of carbohydrates, proteins, and fat, plus phytochemical-rich fruits and vegetables to help the healing process that the body goes through after childbirth. And, if you're a breast-feeding mom, it provides all the nutrients necessary for successful breast-feeding and a thriving baby. Many doctors refer new mothers to me for the *Body After Baby* plan—it's safe and it works. But if you have any concerns, show the plan to your health-care provider before you begin.

Q | *Can I expect to lose weight on the* Body After Baby *plan even if I don't begin right after delivery?*
A | Yes, definitely! While it's true that it's easier to lose weight in the first thirty

days after childbirth, the *Body After Baby* plan will work for you, even if you had your baby several months ago. Your weight loss probably will be slower and you may want to increase the intensity of the exercises if you're feeling up to it. Remember, this healthy eating approach is an appropriate, balanced program that can be followed by adults at any time. Modify your portion sizes to meet your personal circumstances. And keep in mind that the plan is designed for nursing mothers. If you're not nursing, make the adjustments indicated on each day of the plan.

Q | *I'm a vegetarian. Can I use the* Body After Baby *plan?*
A | Yes, I have designed a 15-day *Body After Baby* plan just for vegetarians, which can be repeated over and over again. These menus provide the essential nutrients that are available from the nonvegetarian recipes on the *Body After Baby* plan. Vegetarians need to be aware of their iron and calcium intake, so you can be confident that the veggie alternatives I've included for you are rich with these important minerals. I'm an advocate of eating many plant foods, so I include many vegetarian meals in the regular *Body After Baby* plan. The *Body After Baby* plan combines proteins derived from plants that complement each other so that together they provide a complete set of amino acids that the body recognizes as complete proteins. Whole grains combined with legumes, such as brown rice and lentils, are an example of such a combination.

Q | *I think I'll lose more weight on a high-protein diet. Can I adjust the* Body After Baby *plan to be higher in protein?*
A | The *Body After Baby* plan contains plenty of protein for postpartum moms. In fact, about 25 percent of the calories are derived from various protein sources. By eating foods that have the proper balance of the macronutrients (proteins, fats, and complex carbohydrates), you also get a nutritious supply of micronutrients (vitamins, minerals, and phytochemicals) that are important to a healthy diet. Although you may think you'll lose more weight on a high-protein diet, you'll be risking your health, and, if you're breast-feeding, you'll be taking the chance that your milk supply won't be adequate. In addition, more protein will just put an increased load on your kidneys and may interfere with the favorable hormonal responses that will help you lose your weight naturally and quickly. High-protein diets are typically high-fat diets as well, since most animal proteins contain fat, some more than others. Diets high in animal fat are not recommended for anyone, but

especially not for postpartum moms. You need not get any more than 20–25 percent of your daily calories from fat and most of it should be monounsaturated fats (olive, peanut, and canola oils, as well as avocados and most nuts), polyunsaturated fats (vegetable oils such as safflower, corn, sunflower, and soy) and omega-3 fatty acids (in fatty, cold-water fish such as salmon, mackerel, and herring [check with your fishmonger about the risk of contaminants], walnuts, soybeans, pumpkin seeds, and flaxseed).

Q | *Which foods can help me sleep better?*

A | From a purely physical standpoint, high-carbohydrate foods produce a calming effect on the body. From a psychological standpoint, the food that calms you most just might be chocolate. I know it is for me, despite the minimal caffeine it contains. It just seems to help me feel right in life—and I know many, many other women experience the same effects! Try having 1 ounce of chocolate before bedtime and see if that doesn't help. Another favorite sleep-inducing food is Brown Rice Pudding. (Cook ¼ cup brown rice in ½ cup fat-free milk with a pinch of brown sugar and cinnamon over low heat until the milk is absorbed and the rice is soft and creamy.) Both the brown rice and milk are excellent sources of tryptophan, an essential amino acid that stimulates the production of serotonin, which in turn helps us to relax. You'll also find tryptophan in snacks like cottage cheese, soy nuts, sesame seeds, whole grains, bananas, fish, poultry, and turnips.

Q | *When am I supposed to find time to exercise? I'm always with the baby.*

A | During the postpartum period, your infant is the focus of your attention. As soon as you start the *Body After Baby* plan, I encourage you to include your child in as much of your program as you can. Let your baby see you while you take those few minutes to "work the plan" and experience the movements—you'll still be sharing space with the baby and doing something that will benefit both of you! The *Body After Baby* plan is designed to incorporate exercise into your day conveniently. You don't have to block out a 30- or 60-minute period of time just for exercise. Instead, you can perform the movements while you're cooking dinner, while you're talking on the phone, even while you're lying in bed or just having a good time playing with your baby. Plus, I've designed several Mom and Baby movements, so you and your baby can start a healthy habit of exercising together.

Q | *What's the right weight goal for me?*

A | You can use BMI (body mass index) as a way to determine your best weight. BMI indicates the percentage of your body weight that is fat. A percentage under 25 percent is desirable. Between 25 and 29.9 percent is considered overweight. And 30 percent or greater is considered obese. Use the chart on page 347 to find a range of weights that is healthy for your height. Try not to get overly focused on meeting a particular weight goal. It's much healthier to aim for lean and fit, since being "overfat" is what harms your health. Your favorite pair of jeans can be a good measure. And you should always try to set and reset fitness goals so you are always challenging yourself to get stronger.

Q | *Can I mix up the meals and menus on the* Body After Baby *plan? Can I leave out certain foods?*

A | Each day of the *Body After Baby* plan is carefully divided into three Super phases and each is balanced to provide the nutrients you need to maintain your health and energy while losing weight. If you mix up the meals on various menus, you may not get all the important nutrients that a new mom needs. So my suggestion is to eliminate the days you don't like if you really don't like them, and replace each with another day's complete menu, as long as it's in the same phase of the plan.

Q | *How much water do I need to drink to produce adequate breast milk?*

A | I recommend that you drink a minimum of 2.5 quarts (80 ounces) of water a day while you're breast-feeding. That's approximately one 8-ounce glass every hour for ten hours, and more is better for a breast-feeding mom. You may want to drink those glasses of water earlier in the day rather than near bedtime, so you don't have to get up frequently during the night. However, if you're breast-feeding, keep a covered glass of water near your bed to drink during those late-night feedings.

Q | *Will what I eat help my anemia?*

A | You'll want to consult your health-care professional if you suspect you are anemic. Depending on the severity of your anemia, you may need to take iron supplements in addition to eating the iron-rich meals in the *Body After Baby* menus. However, the right foods will go a long way toward fortifying your blood. Both animal and plant food sources can be great sources for iron. Some of my favorites include ¼ cup canned clams, 1 cup Swiss chard, 1 cup cooked quinoa, 1 tablespoon blackstrap molasses, 1 cup soybeans, or a serving of iron-fortified whole-grain cereal. If you have been diagnosed with anemia, your health-care professional will prescribe an appropriate supplement. Discuss the *Body After Baby* plan so he or she knows that your meals have sources of iron.

Q | *How can what I eat help with postpartum depression?*
A | Many foods—such as dark chocolate or a plain baked potato—contain nutrients and phytochemical compounds that trigger hormones that promote an elevated mood. While many of the food/mood ties are well documented, if you think you are depressed, you should also consult with your health-care professional for help.

Q | *If I'm not breast-feeding, should I eat smaller portions?*
A | Yes, to lose weight you'll need to, and that's why I've included a modification that you can make each day to the plan. You need 500–600 fewer calories each day (on the average), but the same, nutritionally balanced meals. It's important that you keep your diet as balanced as possible because tending to an infant is a big job that keeps you on call twenty-four hours a day.

Q | *Will a low-fat diet affect my breast-feeding?*
A | The *Body After Baby* plan contains plenty of healthy fats to meet the needs of a postpartum mom. Very low-fat diets are never recommended because fat plays an important role in your diet, aiding in the transport and absorption of fat-soluble vitamins and nutrients, maintaining body temperature, and cushioning vital organs. Dietary fat provides two essential fatty acids, omega-3 and omega-6, which are necessary for a variety of physiological processes. A diet that contains 20–25 percent of its calories from healthy fat is within the recommendations of the American Heart Association, American Cancer Society, and American Diabetes Association, as well as the FDA.

Q | *Will the foods on the* Body After Baby *plan cause gas or colic in my baby?*
A | As a nursing mom, you can eat just about any foods you want without worrying about the effect on your breast milk—as long as those foods are nutritious. Some of my *Body After Baby* moms worry that what they eat will pass into their

milk and cause their babies to have colic and gas. The concerns about colic are generally unfounded. Most research shows that colic is not caused by the food mothers ingest. But babies can get gassy from certain foods that typically cause gas in adults and older children: beans, cruciferous vegetables, and dairy products. These bouts are generally short, whereas colic is a chronic condition that occurs daily, striking at about the same time each day, and usually lasts for several weeks. If your child repeatedly gets symptoms that indicate discomfort every time you eat a certain food, it makes sense to stop eating the food. But don't avoid foods that are good for you out of fear that they might cause a problem. In most cases, they won't.

It's not very common, but some babies are allergic to dairy products. Symptoms will include diarrhea, rash, irritability, and gas. If you think your baby is allergic to cow's-milk products, discuss it with your pediatrician, and if he or she agrees, cut out all dairy products from your diet for two weeks. Add them back one at a time and see how your baby reacts. During this time, increase your intake of other calcium-rich foods, such as orange juice that's fortified with calcium, fish with edible bones, bok choy, broccoli, kale, and other dark leafy greens. Your health-care professional may suggest a calcium supplement for you. Meanwhile, when you add a dairy product back into your diet, observe the reactions your baby has and follow the clues to learn what your little one can tolerate.

Q | *How can I adapt the* Body After Baby *plan to provide enough food for me to nurse my twins?*

A | Moms who are breast-feeding more than one child need additional nutrients. You should increase your daily caloric intake by about 500–600 calories per additional infant. That means 500–600 calories for twins and 1,000–1,200 calories for triplets. In most cases that means doubling or tripling the portion size of your meal at breakfast, lunch, and dinner. Or you may choose to turn your snacks into full-sized meals, adding a main course, perhaps leftovers from the night before. Increasing your fat-free milk intake at meals is another healthy way to increase your caloric intake. Be sure to drink water, milk, or 6 oz. fruit juice (which you can dilute with sparkling water) whenever you nurse.

Q | *Can my family eat the same food I eat?*

A | You bet—and they'll love it! Keep it simple and make enough for everyone to enjoy together. You can simply multiply the ingredients based on the number of servings you need for your family. My children love my Pasta with Turkey Meat Sauce, Rockin' Moroccan Sirloin Roast, Wild Berry Smoothies, and, of course, the Chocolate Chip Spice Cake. They'll even confess to liking salmon if I follow the Grilled Salmon with Jicama Orange Salsa recipe!

Q | *I'm lactose intolerant. Can I still use the* Body After Baby *plan since it has lots of milk and cheese?*

A | There are many dairy-free alternatives at the market that can help you adapt the *Body After Baby* recipes to suit your dietary needs. In many recipes you can just substitute an equal amount of the nondairy option. Other good sources of calcium include fish, tofu (calcium is used as part of the coagulant in the tofu-making process), and dark leafy greens such as kale, turnip greens, broccoli, mustard greens, and Brussels sprouts.

Q | *Can I still drink coffee and alcohol?*

A | Both can transfer through your breast milk to your infant, so neither is recommended. Caffeine can accumulate in your baby's system and cause nervousness, poor breast-feeding, and, of course, problems sleeping. The American Academy of Pediatrics recommends that you drink no more than one cup of coffee a day. If you can, try to eliminate that cup too while you're breast-feeding, since it can interfere with your sleep or your baby's. If you can't give up your coffee, consider decaf or half-caf coffee instead of the "fully loaded" version. Alcohol also passes into the baby's system through your milk. If you choose to have a glass of wine, which I do not recommend during the breast-feeding phase of the postpartum period, have it after you nurse the baby, not before, says the American Academy of Pediatrics.

Q | *I keep hearing about whole grains. What does it mean?*

A | A whole grain contains of all three parts of the grain seed, which is also known as the kernel. The three parts of the kernel are the bran, germ, and endosperm. All are rich with nutrients. You can recognize whole-grain products by the description in the ingredient listing, which will include the word "whole" when it's a wheat product. Rye, brown rice, barley, oats, quinoa, and millet are examples of whole grains that are not wheat.

Q | *My husband gained sympathy weight while I was pregnant. Can he follow the* Body After Baby *plan?*

A | Yes. Social support is very helpful for anyone trying to stick to a "new" regimen. My client Linda started the *Body After Baby* plan with her husband, Jay, since they both gained weight during her pregnancy. Linda started right after their baby Emma was born and lost twelve pounds in the first two weeks. Then, they both started eating *Body After Baby* meals. She continued to lose and Jay was amazed that his "pregnancy weight" also started to drop off. After four weeks they both had lost seven pounds—a total of nineteen pounds for Linda in the first month. Keep in mind, though, that the size of your husband's portions may need to be adjusted, depending on his height, weight, activity level, and weight goal. In general, however, plan that your husband's will be 1½ times the size of yours.

Q | *I am tired all the time. What foods will make me feel more energetic?*

A | A balance of protein, fats, and carbohydrates provides optimal energy, but the body gets its immediate energy from complex carbohydrates (see chapter 3). Make sure you're consuming enough water, too, as dehydration often leads to fatigue, and we don't always recognize when we're dehydrated!

Q | *Will the* Body After Baby *plan make me feel gassy or bloated? Will my baby suffer since I'm breast-feeding?*

A | Your gas is not transferred to your baby; however, babies do get gas from some of the same foods that produce gas in adults. To ease your discomfort, drink plenty of water to keep your digestive tract moving, and make sure you're not swallowing too much air when you chew. Eat slowly, too, as eating too fast can cause gas. And surprisingly, even chewing gum can make you feel gassy, since air enters through your mouth while chewing (many of the sugar-free gum products contain sweeteners like sorbitol, which cause gas).

Q | *How much exercise is too much exercise?*

A | Your body will tell you if you're overdoing it. But muscle soreness is different from pain, so don't be afraid to exert yourself to the point that you can feel the muscles working. An effective workout program is progressively more difficult over time, and it demands that your muscles work harder as you get stronger.

Q | *Will the plan still work if I just walk and I don't do all the daily exercises?*

A | Walking is a great way to exercise and share time with the baby. Your muscles also need conditioning, though, and simply walking won't accomplish that important conditioning by itself. Try to incorporate the movements that are explained in the daily Movement Focus section of the *Body After Baby* plan—you'll be glad that you did, and your muscle tone and physique will improve as a result.

Q | *Sure, celebrities succeed because they've got somebody to cook for them. I have to cook all these recipes myself. When will I have time?*

A | The *Body After Baby* plan emphasizes meals that are quick and simple to prepare. Many of them can be made in advance. For example, you'll notice that there are just three soups—that's so you can make one batch, freeze the extra servings, and enjoy the soup again later in the plan. If you follow the recipes and have extra servings of other items left over, you can use the storage instructions that accompany the recipes as a guide to determine which can be frozen and/or how long they can be stored in the refrigerator. Also, many of the ingredients can be purchased already chopped, sliced, or diced, either fresh or frozen. You could try asking a friend or family member to help you out with some of the preparation or shopping, in lieu of a baby gift, but if no one is available to help you and you need to save time, you can select the days of the plan within each phase that fit your needs best, and just repeat them more often. You'll miss some of the variety and nutritional benefits of the different foods, but the daily plans are balanced and can be interchanged as needed. Feel free to e-mail me at **jkeller@nutrifitonline.com** if you have any questions about the menus or recipes. I'd be pleased to hear from you and happy to help!

movements

for mom and baby

BONDING WITH YOUR BABY happens whenever you do things together, not just while you're feeding the baby or singing lullabies. You can have quality time with your baby while walking, for example. You can also do exercises with your baby at your side, in your arms, or in a baby carrier. I've taught these "Mommy and me" exercises for years. I show moms how to make exercising with their babies something to really look forward to as a fun part of each day. When my first baby, Alexandra, was two days old, I was marching in place while holding her. During the first ten days after delivery, I found ways to stretch my entire body and not be away from her for a moment. It wasn't long before I was pushing her around the block in the stroller, then, when I felt strong enough, I was walking three miles a day with her strapped in a Snugli! I felt great and the weight was dropping off naturally and easily.

When I talk to experts about the effects of exercise for new moms, they all stress the importance of regular physical activity. Consider what Cindy S. Moskovic, MSW, the director of the Iris Cantor–UCLA Women's Health Education & Resource Center, has to say: "Research has shown that exercise can improve the mood of new moms. Exercise can also increase energy and help improve sleep. These factors are vital to a new mom's ability to manage stress in the weeks and months following childbirth. New moms who engaged in regular, vigorous activity have been shown to be more likely to socialize and participate in hobbies. Perhaps most importantly, regular exercise can promote feelings of empowerment, which can positively impact the new mom's self-esteem."

Walk with Your Baby

Why walk? "Walking is man's best medicine," said the Greek physician Hippocrates, some twenty-five hundred years ago (and I'm sure he meant to say "woman's," too). We now know that walking benefits everyone by helping to lower blood pressure, reduce levels of bad cholesterol, slow bone loss from osteoporosis, and reduce the risk of heart disease. For new moms, walking can also ease back pain, improve muscle tone, enhance stamina, increase energy, and reduce appetite.

Walking with your baby has benefits that go way beyond the physical, however. Walking is a way to reconnect with the world. So many new moms have told me that they've forgotten how to converse with adults after a few weeks of being home with their babies. Walking in the neighborhood or in a park ends that isolation. You meet other moms—you can't help it! And those walks allow you to develop new friendships with other moms who may be as interested in adult camaraderie as you are. You've got the common bond of experiencing new motherhood. And walking is a social tool that's not only good for you, but it's great for your baby as well.

The big plus is that walking burns almost as many calories as jogging. Start walking with your baby as soon as you feel able, and gradually build up the number of steps you walk each day. While you're walking, remember to take deep, regular breaths, keep your back straight, your stride long and smooth, and let your arms swing naturally at your sides if you have your baby in a wearable carrier. If you're pushing the baby in a stroller, keep your posture in mind, so you don't become hunched over. Wear loose, comfortable clothing, a bra that provides plenty of support, and shoes that do, too.

I encourage you to use a pedometer and aim for 10,000 steps a day, which is the number of steps we should take each day to maintain health, according to the U.S. Surgeon General. You may not be able to achieve that goal right away, but you'll be amazed at how quickly the steps add up when you couple going for walks with the baby with tending to the baby at home, doing some light housework, going to the market, and running errands. Make certain that before you begin your longer walks that you've had some water to drink and don't forget to take some water with you. Warm up by doing some of the gentle stretches you've learned on the *Body After Baby* plan. Walk slowly at first, then try to speed up your pace in the middle of your walk—even break a sweat if you can. And when you're ready to stop, cool down slowly.

POSTURE IS ESPECIALLY IMPORTANT NOW

The more you use your muscles to stand, sit, and walk properly, the stronger those muscles that support your body will become. I know that sounds easy—and it is—but after giving birth, your muscles need some reminders. Walking with your baby in a stroller or in a wearable baby carrier can wreak havoc on your posture—your shoulders round, you start to slump, and your balance is off. So whenever you're moving, you must be conscious of your posture and work to strengthen your support muscles.

Part of the problem is that for the last twelve weeks of pregnancy, your back swayed to balance the belly that was expanding in front of you. Your pelvis widened as it prepared for delivery. Your feet turned out to give you a broader base of support. For the last several months, your center of balance changed as baby grew inside of you. A wearable baby carrier or pushing a stroller can reinforce that bad posture. So now it's time to retrain your muscles to support the new, lighter you.

You can work on your posture whether you are out walking or working in the house. Here's an easy posture exercise. Do it right now! Stand up, roll your shoulders down and back, and lift your chest (pretend your chest is your shield, a coat of armor, protecting your heart), tightening your stomach muscles as you stand. Lace your fingers behind your back and turn your palms down. Consciously walk in a straight line for three minutes, concentrating on maintaining this healthy posture. Do this as many times during the day as you can. In a couple of weeks you'll find that your posture has improved dramatically and that standing and walking with a straight back has become a habit.

When you're carrying your baby, try to keep your stomach muscles contracted. This will help support your back and it will also help to strengthen your abs at the same time. Be sure to keep your shoulders relaxed, too. When you feel your shoulders getting tense, roll them forward and then roll them backward, one at a time. Switch the baby from one side to the other as you do this. Most moms mistakenly get in the habit of carrying their infants on one hip or the other all the time. This is not only bad for your back; it also causes you to lift that hip, throwing off your balanced posture.

Before and after a walk do some of the gentle movements from the plan. The Shoulder Roll, Chest Stretch, and Neck Press are all excellent exercises for strengthening muscles that control your posture. Likewise, the abdominal and back muscles work to align your whole body, so do the Partial Sit-ups and Reach and Crunches whenever you can after a walk.

Check your posture from the ground up. If your body is properly aligned, you should be able to answer yes to each question.

- Are your knees relaxed?
- Are your buttocks tucked?
- Are your stomach muscles comfortably contracted?
- Is your chest up?
- Are your shoulders down, slightly back, and even with each other?
- Are you looking straight ahead, so your chin is neither tilted down nor up?
- Is your head directly over your shoulders?

When you walk you should maintain a comfortable posture and relaxed gait. You should be able to answer yes to each question:

- Do you step on your heel and roll to your toe?
- Is your stomach tight?
- Is your chest forward, like a shield in front of your heart?
- Do your arms swing gently by your sides?
- Do you step lightly on your feet?

MOM AND BABY MOVEMENTS

The movements in this chapter are exercises that you will love to do with your baby because they're enjoyable and they're easy. As long as you approach postpartum exercise wisely and have your ob-gyn's approval, there's no reason you can't do simple exercises almost immediately. The movements I describe here coincide with each phase of the *Body After Baby* plan, but you can start them whenever you want to. These exercises are so easy that you don't need to go to a class, but if you like to socialize with other moms, a "Mommy and me" program is a great place to find some new workout and walking buddies.

Swing and Smile

❋ Kneel on your exercise mat and sit back on your heels, with your baby in front of you.

❋ With your face about 12 inches from the baby's face, move your head from side to side, smiling and talking as you move. This will help to strengthen your neck muscles and baby's, since the baby will follow your eyes and your voice as you move!

❋ Practice good posture while doing this simple movement, and keep your stomach muscles contracted. You can even do Kegels!

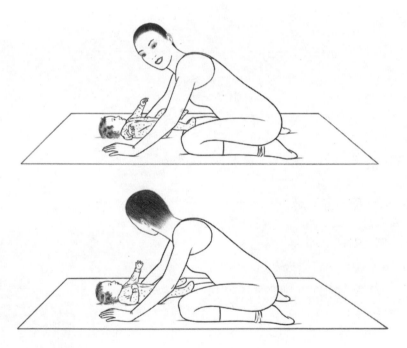

Cat Stretch

❋ Lay your baby on his or her back on a blanket.

❋ Kneel in front of the baby and then put your hands flat on the mat about 2 feet in front of your knees, directly under your shoulders. The baby is now underneath you. Keep your stomach taut and your back in a straight horizontal line.

✤ Inhale deeply and arch your back, just like a cat. Tighten your abdominals as you arch, holding the stretch for three seconds.

✤ Release, slowly exhaling as you return to the starting position. Be sure not to let your stomach sag or your back sway.

✤ Repeat eight times. The baby will enjoy watching you move! If it's long enough, you can let your hair fall forward and tickle your baby with it, if that entertains your little one! Or try meowing like a cat and watch your baby laugh or smile.

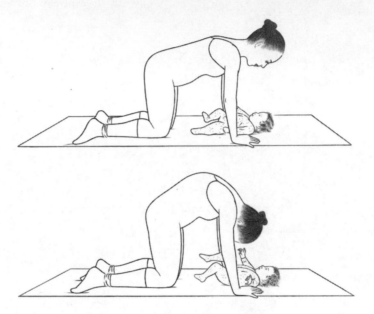

Seated Calf Raises

✤ Sit on a straight-backed chair with your stomach muscles contracted, your back straight, and your shoulders relaxed.

✤ Cradle your infant, supporting his or her neck, back, and bottom.

✤ Raise your heels so your weight is on the balls of your feet and hold for the count of three.

✤ Now lower your heels, pressing them firmly into the floor!

✤ Repeat fifteen times.

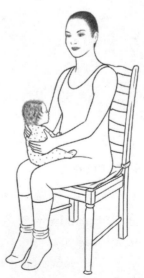

Thigh Firmers

❋ With your feet flat on the floor, sit tall but comfortably on a straight-backed chair, holding your baby securely.

❋ Stretch the other leg out to the side.

❋ With thigh muscles contracted, bring your leg back to the starting position.

❋ Repeat ten times.

❋ Switch position of baby to the other leg, and repeat the leg movement using the opposite leg.

❋ Repeat ten times.

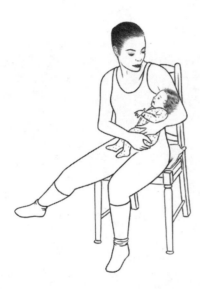

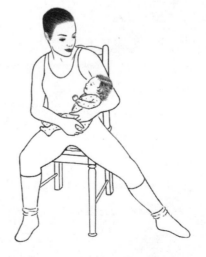

March in Place with Baby

Since walking is one of the best exercises that you can do with your baby, get in shape now for longer walks later. Strap the baby comfortably into a wearable baby carrier, so your hands are free. March in place for five minutes, lifting your knees as high as you can. It's a great time to sing and tickle your child so he or she knows it's a happy time. Do this every day and increase the duration by two minutes every three days.

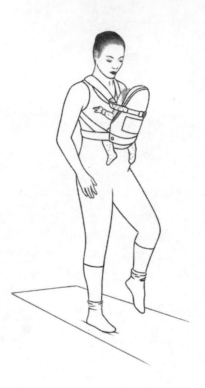

Lying Leg Lifts

❋ With your baby lying on a blanket in front of you, lie on your right side with your shoulders and hips in a straight line, your left leg extended straight over your right, keeping your right leg bent back at the knee for extra support. Support your head with your right arm and use your left arm for support and balance if needed.

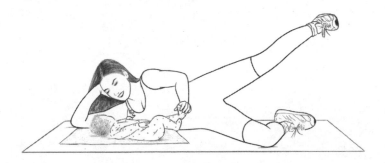

❋ Contract your abdominal muscles firmly and lift your left leg toward the ceiling, keeping your foot flexed and your knee forward (not rotated upward toward the ceiling!). As you lift your leg, gently lift your baby's leg too.

❋ Lower your leg and lower the baby's.

❋ Repeat ten times with each leg. When you switch sides, be sure to keep the baby in front of you, so you can easily lift his or her legs.

Mama Squat

❋ Standing with your feet about shoulder-width apart and toes pointed straight ahead, cradle your baby in both arms, supporting his or her neck, spine, and bottom.

❋ Slowly bend your knees until your thighs are parallel to the floor. As you squat, hold the baby close to you as you slowly inhale.

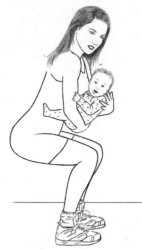

❋ Now straighten your legs, exhaling as you return to your starting position.

❋ Repeat five times.

Baby Lifts

❋ Sitting straight in a chair, hold your baby on your knees with one hand supporting the baby's neck and the other hand under the baby's bottom.

❋ With slow, controlled movements, lift and lower the baby, keeping your arms extended in front of you.

❋ Repeat ten times. Keep your eyes focused on the baby—he or she will love it!

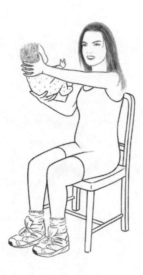 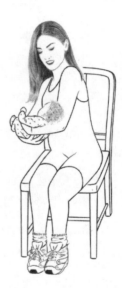

Waist Twists

❋ Sit in a straight-backed chair with your feet flat on the floor and cradle the baby in your arms, making sure the baby's neck, back, and bottom are completely supported.

❋ Gently twist from side to side, moving through one full range of motion without slouching. Contract your abdominals tightly as you twist from the waist.

❋ Complete a set of ten twists, or as many as the baby enjoys. My son, Adam, loved this movement more than all the others. Of course, now he denies it—what a typical teenager!

Pec Press

🌸 Position the baby securely in a bouncer on a table or countertop.

🌸 Stand facing the baby, about an arm's length away.

🌸 Extend your arms directly in front of you at chest height, with your elbows slightly bent and your wrists flexed.

🌸 Bring the heels of your hands together in front of you, while you keep your chest muscles taut; this will create a strengthening resistance.

🌸 Now, slowly open your arms wide.

🌸 Repeat ten times. You can sing a favorite song to baby as you do this! Be sure to maintain eye contact with baby throughout the exercise. After you've done your set, you can exercise the baby's chest muscles by moving his or her arms, too!

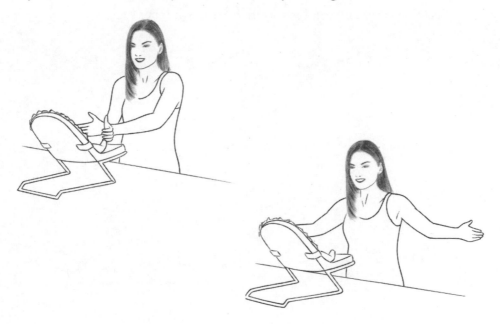

Modified Push-ups

❁ With the baby on a blanket on the floor next to you, support your body on your hands and knees. Yes, those same "girl" push-ups you did in high school.

❁ Slowly lower your upper body by bending your elbows out to the sides.

❁ Bring your chest toward the floor, keeping your back in a straight line.

❁ Push up by straightening your arms and returning to the starting position. Keep your tummy muscles tight through the entire motion.

❁ As you press down, you can tell your baby, "Here comes Mommy!" As you press up, say, "Here goes Mommy!"

❁ Repeat five times and comfortably increase the number each day.

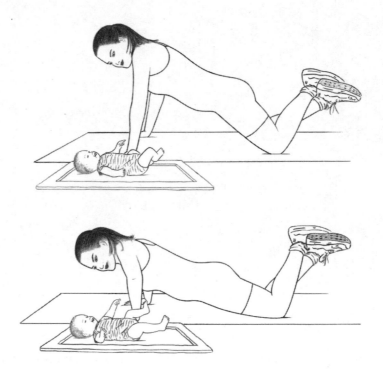

Torso Stretch

❋ With the baby in a bouncer facing you, lie on your stomach on a mat with your legs slightly apart and toes pointed.

❋ Press your hands into the mat and lift your upper body, shifting your weight onto your forearms as you press up. Keep your hip bones on the mat. As you stretch your abdomen and torso, you strengthen your spine. Open and close your eyes, playing peekaboo with the baby.

❋ Return to starting position.

❋ Repeat the stretch ten times, playing peekaboo each time.

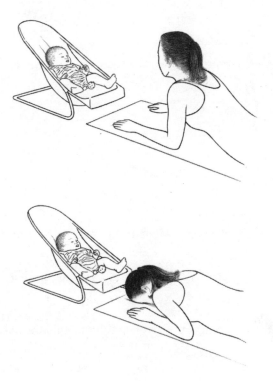

Tush Tightener

❋ Lying on your stomach, with the baby in front of you on a blanket, rest on your forearms so you are looking at your baby. Your legs should be shoulder-width apart.

❋ Squeeze your buttocks as you bring your heels together, tightening your buttocks. Hold for the count of three.

✽ Repeat ten times. After you've done your set, try to gently bring the baby's legs apart and together in a similar movement.

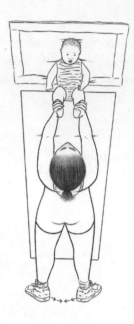 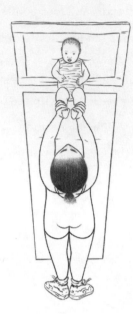

Lying Runner's Stretch

✽ With the baby on a blanket in front of you, lie on your side (your hips should be in line with each other). Bend your top leg at the knee, so your heel comes close to your buttocks.

✽ Grasp the top of your foot with your hand, pulling the heel closer to your buttocks.

✽ Hold the stretch for the count of ten, release, and tickle the baby.

✽ Repeat three times on each side.

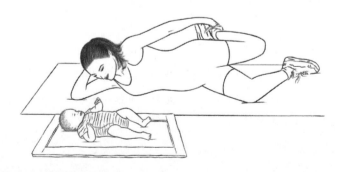

Bent-over Baby Raises

This is a modified version of a traditional weight-lifting exercise called "Good Morning." It's much more fun to lift your baby than a barbell—you'll see!

❁ Start with baby lying on a chair in front of you.

❁ As you face baby on the chair, bend from the waist, pick up baby, tighten your abdominal muscles, and stand up straight, cradling baby to your chest.

❁ Return to starting position.

❁ Repeat this bending and lifting action ten times, keeping the muscles contracted, without relaxing between each lift.

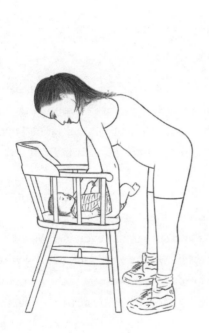
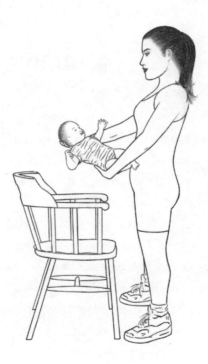

making good health a family matter

A HEALTHY BODY heals quickly after the birth of a baby. That's nature's way of making moms strong and able to take care of young ones as soon as possible. But you give nature a hand by taking care of yourself, too. That's why carefully planned food and exercise are both so important to the *Body After Baby* plan.

I want to encourage you to make healthy eating and exercise more than just a part of your life, but also part of your entire family's life. It's up to us, as parents, to help our children practice healthy eating habits and get regular exercise. We establish a pattern for our kids to follow by what we say, what we do, and, yes, by what we teach them (note: *teach,* not *preach*). If we practice what we teach, they will follow our lead. We are their role models. If we eat right and are physically active, the odds are far better that our children will make the same healthy decisions. And by making these choices, each child will find it easier to maintain an appropriate weight—and have a great attitude about daily exercise.

U.S. Department of Health and Human Services research shows that 16 percent of the children and teens in America are overweight. What does that mean for a child? Socially, it means it's harder to keep up with other kids, that when they're in school they don't look forward to recess (they often dread it), and they're more prone to be teased and bullied by other kids. On a health level it means that they're

food, exercise, and family dynamics

THE benefits of adopting a sound nutrition and exercise program after your pregnancy go far beyond benefiting just you. Your new baby benefits, as do all the members of your immediate family. After delivery, there can be wide fluctuations in a variety of hormones that can make you susceptible to mood swings for many weeks. With all of the responsibilities inherent to caring for your new baby, it is difficult to find time to exercise—but if you can, you can help keep your mood stable. When you exercise at about 60–70 percent of your maximum heart rate (that rate can vary depending on your age, etc., so check with your doctor to establish yours) for as little as twenty minutes a day, your body will release endorphins, hormones that can help to moderate mood. A happier mom affects the whole family. If you are also following a healthy eating regimen, you help your family to have more energy to exercise more efficiently, which means you all will sleep better—and that includes the baby, a big plus! All of this adds up to happier family dynamics. Finally, if you set the important pattern of eating well *together* at dinner in the earliest stages of your family life, you establish a family tradition that will have great meaning as your family matures. Research has shown, time and again, that the family that has a pattern of eating dinner together benefits both physically and emotionally. The family dinnertime should be sacrosanct.

—SHARI KAHANE, M.D., R.N.
Family Practice and Emergency Medicine,
San Fernando Valley, California

prone to Type 2 diabetes, a disease that was once rare in children. Now as many as 45 percent of the newly diagnosed cases of childhood diabetes are Type 2, which often can be prevented by proper diet and regular exercise. And research clearly shows that children who are overweight tend to become overweight or obese adults.

What can you do? If you want your family to be healthy, make it happen. Moms have that power. It's no surprise that the impact you have on your children's eating and exercising habits begins immediately. Why wait until they're older to instill good habits? Everything you do *right now* gets absorbed by your children. Every smile. Every hug. Every walk. Every food choice. A study at Pennsylvania State University showed that moms who ate more fruits and vegetables passed the same habits on to their daughters. Similarly, a British study confirmed that a child's consumption of fruits and vegetables was not just based on whether or not he or she liked them, but by how much his or her mother knows about the nutritional value of these healthy foods, her attitude about healthy eating, and her own consumption

get out and walk!

"TAKE two aerobics classes and call me in the morning" may now be shown to be an antidote for the baby blues. Clinical research studies have concluded that a strong link exists between exercise and easing postpartum depression. I have found that exercise is more effective for the long-term control of depression than any psychotropic drug. I urge mothers to get outdoors and walk, not just to lift their own spirits, but to create an active bonding time for the whole family—siblings, parents, family pets. This allows the entire family, especially the new mom, to get out of the house and expand each other's appreciation of their new family and their environment. Involve the other children with the new baby. Run together. Play games. This is a great way to get the family to be active together and watch everyone's spirits soar!

—LINDA STEELE, PH.D.
Clinical psychologist and therapeutic life coach,
West Los Angeles and Santa Monica, California

of fruits and vegetables. If you place a high value on healthy foods, make them available, and eat them, so will your child.

The same goes for exercise. From infancy through the toddler years, your child will learn that physical activity is a priority if you make it a priority. Whether being pushed in a stroller as an infant or playing in the park as a toddler, your child gets into the mode of outdoor activity. And as your child gets older, how about a game of catch in the yard or a set of Ping-Pong? Participate in team sports with your kids, even if that means simply being there to root for them and their teams on the weekends. My daughter, Alexandra, chose soccer as her team sport. Now she and her brother, Adam, are into Kendo and have just begun to learn how to surf. They're not sports enthusiasts by any means, but we support their efforts by encouraging them to try different things. Parental encouragement and involvement raises children's interest, enthusiasm, and self-esteem.

My husband, Phil, has always been very supportive of my exercise time. Even though we work long hours, he recognizes my need to have time each day "just for me." When the kids were small, Phil would play with them in the living room or take them out for a walk while I decompressed. Truthfully, some of our best times have been, and continue to be, spent outdoors doing things together. Even though our children aren't always "super excited" initially, they end up enjoying a family hike or other physically active family together-time. Phil and I make it a point to initiate active—not passive—family activities on a regular basis. And we all look forward to sharing that time together.

Like you, there was a time when I, too, felt overwhelmed and uncertain about how to manage my responsibilities as a new mom. I don't know a new mother who hasn't had those feelings. My goal with the *Body After Baby* plan was to create a plan that would alleviate two major concerns: your nutritional health and your body image. The *Body After Baby* plan gives you an easy-to-follow blueprint for how to manage these concerns successfully. It's a step-by-step way for you to lose your baby weight; you don't have to second-guess anything, you just follow the plan. And the best part about it is that the plan is "new mom-tested"—it's worked for hundreds of *Body After Baby* moms.

Enjoy the *Body After Baby* plan and, most of all, enjoy your wonderful new family.

recipes

A Note About Recipes

The nutritional values listed for each recipe are specific to the serving size indicated. If you are preparing meals for more than one person, you may want to adjust the serving size. In all cases, please follow the meal plan and enjoy the serving size or number of servings indicated in your meal plan in chapter 4.

Most of the recipes include a list of beneficial nutrients. An "excellent source" of a micronutrient is defined as having more than 20 percent of the Reference Daily Intake (RDI) or Daily Reference Value (DRV). A "good source" of a micronutrient is defined as having between 10-19 percent of the RDI or DRV.

aegean cod

SERVINGS: 6

INGREDIENTS

Extra-virgin olive oil cooking spray

2 lbs. (6 fillets) cod

2 plum tomatoes, chopped

1 small onion, finely chopped

1 Tbsp. NutriFit Mediterranean Salt Free Spice Blend

1 Tbsp. lemon juice

1 Tbsp. extra-virgin olive oil

DIRECTIONS

Note: For each tablespoon of the NutriFit Mediterranean Salt Free Spice Blend you may substitute: 1 tsp. oregano, 1 tsp. basil, ½ tsp. black pepper, and ½ tsp. garlic powder.

1 Coat a baking pan with cooking spray. Rinse the fish and pat dry with paper towels. Place the fish in the pan.

2 In a small bowl, combine the remaining ingredients. Rub the mixture on the fish. Refrigerate for about 15 minutes.

3 Preheat the oven to 400°F.

4 Bake the fish for about 30 minutes, or until it flakes easily with a fork and is opaque inside.

STORAGE INSTRUCTIONS

Best eaten within 2 days; do not freeze.

NUTRIENT INFORMATION (serving size: 5 oz., or the size of the palm of your hand)
Calories: 195; Protein: 35.2 g; Carbohydrates: 3.8 g; Fat: 3.7 g; Fiber: 0.8 g

OTHER BENEFICIAL NUTRIENTS:
Excellent source of: vitamin A, vitamin C, vitamin B_6
Good source of: folacin

angel food cake

INGREDIENTS

1½ cups egg whites

1½ tsp. cream of tartar

1 Tbsp. lemon juice

1 tsp. vanilla extract

1 cup cake flour, sifted

1 cup granulated sugar

1½ cups powdered sugar, sifted

DIRECTIONS

1 Preheat the oven to 350°F. Separate the eggs, and put the whites in a very clean, deep, glass or stainless steel bowl. Allow the whites to warm to room temperature (after separating) for maximum volume. Refrigerate the yolks for later use.

2 Whip the egg whites until foamy, then add the cream of tartar and whip the mixture until stiff but not dry.

3 Fold in the lemon juice and vanilla. Mix the flour and sugars in a bowl. Sift about ¼ cup of the dry mixture over the batter. Fold in gently, but quickly. Continue until all of the mixture is incorporated, mixing as little as possible to minimize the breakdown of the whites.

4 Pour the batter into an ungreased tube pan. Bake for about 45 minutes, until the top is dry and the side pulls away from the pan.

5 To cool, use an inverted funnel or a soft-drink bottle to invert the pan (cool upside down) if the tube is not high enough to keep the cake above the surface of the cooling rack. Let the cake hang for about 1½ hours, until it is thoroughly set. Remove the cake from the pan before storing.

STORAGE INSTRUCTIONS

Store at room temperature; may be frozen.

NUTRIENT INFORMATION (serving size: 1 slice):
Calories: 73; Protein: 1.7 g; Carbohydrates: 16.4 g; Fat: 0.2 g; Fiber: 0.4 g

artichoke dip

SERVINGS: 10

INGREDIENTS

1 (8-oz.) can artichoke hearts, drained

2 Tbsp. grated onion (optional)

½ cup fat-free ricotta cheese

½ cup fat-free sour cream

8 oz. fat-free cream cheese

¼ cup fat-free mayonnaise

¼ cup grated fat-free Parmesan cheese

⅛ tsp. NutriFit Calypso Salt Free Spice Blend

1 whole round bread (for presentation)

DIRECTIONS

Note: For each teaspoon of the NutriFit Calypso Salt Free Spice Blend you may substitute: ½ tsp. ground chiles, ¼ tsp. ground cumin, ⅛ tsp. black pepper, and ⅛ tsp. garlic powder.

1 Preheat the oven to 350°F.

2 Drain the artichoke hearts, discarding the liquid. In a food processor, coarsely chop the artichokes. Add the onion (optional) and process with three more short bursts. Add the remaining ingredients, except the bread, and process with short bursts just until blended, being careful not to overprocess.

3 Hollow out the center of the bread, reserving the core for bread crumbs or another use. Fill the center of the bread with dip, and bake, uncovered, for 15–20 minutes, or until the dip is hot.

STORAGE INSTRUCTIONS

Refrigerate promptly; do not freeze.

NUTRIENT INFORMATION (serving size: ¼ cup):
Calories: 65; Protein: 7.1 g; Carbohydrates: 7 g; Fat: 0.1 g; Fiber: 0.1 g

OTHER BENEFICIAL NUTRIENTS:
Excellent source of: vitamin A
Good source of: calcium

asian cucumber salad

INGREDIENTS

2 Tbsp. brown sugar

½ cup rice vinegar

2 Tbsp. reduced-sodium soy sauce

¼ tsp. red pepper flakes

2 Tbsp. reduced-sodium vegetable broth

2 Tbsp. minced green onions

6 medium cucumbers, peeled, halved lengthwise, seeded, and thinly sliced

2 tsp. finely chopped roasted peanuts

DIRECTIONS

1 In a small bowl, mix the brown sugar, rice vinegar, soy sauce, red pepper flakes, and vegetable broth.

2 In another bowl, combine the onions, cucumbers, and peanuts. Pour the dressing mixture over. Mix well. Serve immediately or refrigerate.

STORAGE INSTRUCTIONS

Refrigerate promptly; do not freeze.

NUTRIENT INFORMATION (serving size: 1 cup):
Calories: 113; Protein: 4 g; Carbohydrates: 21.4 g; Fat: 1.4 g; Fiber: 3.9 g

OTHER BENEFICIAL NUTRIENTS:
Excellent source of: vitamin A, vitamin C, folacin
Good source of: vitamin B_6, iron, fiber

asparagus broccoli bouquet

SERVINGS: 4

INGREDIENTS

1½ tsp. canola oil

1 medium onion, thinly sliced

1 clove garlic, crushed

¼ tsp. white pepper

¼ tsp. salt

3 cups fresh broccoli flowerets

1 lb. fresh asparagus, trimmed and cut into 1-inch pieces

2 Tbsp. lemon juice

1½ tsp. sugar

DIRECTIONS

1 Heat a large skillet. Add the oil. Cook the onions, garlic, pepper, and salt for about 5 minutes, until the onions are soft.

2 Add the broccoli and asparagus and stir to coat over high heat. Add the lemon juice and sugar. Sauté for about 5 minutes, until the vegetables are tender. Arrange on a plate in the shape of a bouquet of flowers.

STORAGE INSTRUCTIONS

Refrigerate promptly; do not freeze.

NUTRIENT INFORMATION (serving size: 1 cup):
Calories: 77; Protein: 5.3 g; Carbohydrates: 9.8 g; Fat: 2.7 g; Fiber: 3.7 g

OTHER BENEFICIAL NUTRIENTS:
Excellent source of: vitamin A, folacin
Good source of: vitamin B$_6$, fiber

baja-style cod with salsa coulis

SERVINGS: 4

INGREDIENTS

1½ lb. (4 fillets) cod

2 tsp. extra-virgin olive oil

1 Tbsp. lime juice

½ tsp. sea salt

1 tsp. NutriFit Calypso Salt Free Spice Blend

½ cup enchilada sauce

2 Tbsp. fresh salsa, medium spicy

¼ cup fat-free half-and-half

1 Tbsp. minced cilantro

DIRECTIONS

Note: For each teaspoon of the NutriFit Calypso Salt Free Spice Blend you may substitute: ½ tsp. ground chiles, ¼ tsp. ground cumin, ⅛ tsp. black pepper, and ⅛ tsp. garlic powder.

1 Preheat the broiler.

2 Rinse the fish and pat dry. Place the fillets in a single layer in a shallow pan, on a broiler rack. Brush the fish with the olive oil, then drizzle with the lime juice. Sprinkle lightly with the sea salt and the spice blend.

3 Broil the fish about 4 inches from the heat for about 5 minutes, until no longer translucent in the center of the thickest part.

4 While the fish cooks, in a small saucepan, stir the enchilada sauce, salsa, and half-and-half over medium heat for 3–4 minutes.

5 Transfer each fillet to a plate. Spoon some sauce over each portion, then sprinkle with the cilantro.

STORAGE INSTRUCTIONS

Best eaten within 2 days; do not freeze.

NUTRIENT INFORMATION (serving size: 6 oz., about the size of the palm of your hand):
Calories: 180; Protein: 32 g; Carbohydrates: 3 g; Fat: 3.9 g; Fiber: 0.2 g

OTHER BENEFICIAL NUTRIENTS:
Excellent source of: vitamin A, vitamin B_6
Good source of: vitamin C

baked turkey dijon

SERVINGS: 3

INGREDIENTS

1 lb. boneless, skinless turkey breasts

1 Tbsp. Dijon mustard

1 tsp. extra-virgin olive oil

1 clove garlic, minced

2 tsp. lemon juice

1 tsp. NutriFit Lemon Garden Salt Free Spice Blend

DIRECTIONS

Note: For each teaspoon of the NutriFit Lemon Garden Salt Free Spice Blend you may substitute: ¼ tsp. basil, ¼ tsp. marjoram, ¼ tsp. black pepper, and ¼ tsp. dill weed.

1 Preheat the oven to 350°F.

2 Rinse the turkey, pat it dry, and arrange the tenderloins in a single layer in a glass baking dish.

3 In a small bowl, stir together the remaining ingredients and spread the mixture evenly over the top of each piece of turkey.

4 Bake, uncovered, for about 15–20 minutes, or until the turkey is no longer pink in the center.

STORAGE INSTRUCTIONS

Refrigerate promptly; may be frozen.

NUTRIENT INFORMATION (serving size: 5 oz., the size of an audio cassette tape):
Calories: 191; Protein: 37.7 g; Carbohydrates: 1.5 g; Fat: 2.9 g; Fiber: 0.2 g

OTHER BENEFICIAL NUTRIENTS:
Excellent source of: vitamin B_6
Good source of: iron, zinc

balsamic broiled salmon

SERVINGS: 4

INGREDIENTS

Extra-virgin olive oil cooking spray

3 Tbsp. balsamic vinegar

1½ Tbsp. honey

½ tsp. canola oil

4 (4-oz.) salmon fillets (½ inch thick)

DIRECTIONS

1 Preheat the broiler. Spray a baking pan with the cooking spray.

2 In a small bowl, combine the vinegar, honey, and oil; set aside.

3 Wash the salmon and pat dry with paper towels.

4 Place the salmon in the prepared baking pan. Drizzle with half of the vinegar mixture. Place the salmon about 6 inches below heat, and broil, brushing several times with the remaining vinegar mixture, for 8–10 minutes, until just opaque but still moist in the thickest part; cut to test.

STORAGE INSTRUCTIONS

Refrigerate promptly; best not to freeze.

BODY AFTER BABY

NUTRIENT INFORMATION (serving size: 1 fillet):
Calories: 308; Protein: 33.7 g; Carbohydrates: 14.5 g; Fat: 11.6g; Fiber: 0 g

OTHER BENEFICIAL NUTRIENTS:
Excellent source of: vitamin A, vitamin B_6
Good source of: folacin

banana and orange oatmeal

INGREDIENTS

1⅓ cups orange juice

½ tsp. grated orange rind

1⅓ cups quick-cooking rolled oats

1 medium banana, peeled and coarsely chopped

⅛ tsp. NutriFit Certainly Cinnamon Salt Free Spice Blend

1 Tbsp. brown sugar (optional)

½ cup fat-free milk

1 medium orange, peeled and segmented

DIRECTIONS

Note: For each teaspoon of the NutriFit Certainly Cinnamon Salt Free Spice Blend you may substitute: ½ tsp. cinnamon, ¼ tsp. nutmeg, ⅛ tsp. ginger, and ⅛ tsp. cloves.

1 In a nonreactive saucepan, combine the orange juice and rind and bring the mixture to a boil. Stir in the rolled oats, reduce the heat to low, and cook the mixture, covered, for 1 minute. Remove the pan from the heat and let the oatmeal stand, covered, until it has thickened, about 1 minute more.

2 Slice the bananas into the oatmeal and stir to cover the slices so that they do not brown. Add the spice blend and the brown sugar (optional).

3 Spoon the cereal into four individual bowls; add 2 tablespoons of the milk to each bowl and garnish it with one or two of the orange segments. Serve at once.

STORAGE INSTRUCTIONS

Refrigerate promptly; may be frozen.

NUTRIENT INFORMATION (serving size: 1 cup):
Calories: 206; Protein: 6.3 g; Carbohydrates: 41.8 g; Fat: 2g; Fiber: 3.3 g

OTHER BENEFICIAL NUTRIENTS:
Excellent source of: vitamin A, vitamin C, folacin, calcium
Good source of: vitamin B_6, fiber

bell pepper and cheese omelet

SERVINGS: I

INGREDIENTS

1 cup fat-free egg substitute

¼ tsp. NutriFit Calypso Salt
Free Spice Blend

⅛ cup chopped yellow
bell pepper

⅛ cup chopped green
bell pepper

⅛ cup chopped red bell pepper

Canola oil cooking spray

1 oz. shredded reduced-fat
cheddar cheese

DIRECTIONS

Note: For each teaspoon of NutriFit Calypso Salt Free Spice Blend, you may substitute: ½ tsp. ground chiles, ¼ tsp. cumin, ⅛ tsp. black pepper, and ⅛ tsp. garlic powder.

1 In a small bowl, whisk the egg substitute and spice blend together.

2 In a small glass bowl, microwave the peppers, covered, until soft; set aside.

3 Heat a nonstick skillet, then coat with cooking spray and pour the egg mixture into the pan. Cook, allowing the eggs to set and lifting up the edges of the omelet as it forms to allow the liquid to run to the bottom of the skillet. This will allow the bottom of the omelet to cook. Turn when the eggs have set, and add the cheese and the peppers over the bottom half of the omelet. Fold the top half over the cheese, forming a half-moon shape.

4 Serve immediately.

STORAGE INSTRUCTIONS

Refrigerate promptly; do not freeze.

NUTRIENT INFORMATION (serving size: 1 omelet):
Calories: 203; Protein: 34.4 g; Carbohydrates: 6.8 g; Fat: 3.1 g; Fiber: 1.5 g

OTHER BENEFICIAL NUTRIENTS:
Excellent source of: vitamin A, vitamin C, calcium
Good source of: vitamin B_6

black bean salad

INGREDIENTS

3 cups cooked black beans

1 cup chopped tomato

¾ cup diced red bell pepper

¾ cup diced zucchini

½ cup chopped green onions

1 tsp. seeded and minced jalapeño pepper

3 Tbsp. lime juice

3 Tbsp. balsamic vinegar

1 tsp. extra-virgin olive oil

1 Tbsp. NutriFit Calypso Salt Free Spice Blend

DIRECTIONS

Note: For each tablespoon of the NutriFit Calypso Salt Free Spice Blend you may substitute: 1½ tsp. ground chiles, ¾ tsp. cumin, ½ tsp. black pepper, and ¼ tsp. garlic powder.

1 In a large bowl, combine the beans, tomato, bell pepper, zucchini, green onions, and jalapeño pepper; toss gently.

2 In a separate bowl, whisk together the lime juice, balsamic vinegar, olive oil, and spice blend. Pour over the bean mixture; toss gently. Cover and marinate in the refrigerator for up to 8 hours.

STORAGE INSTRUCTIONS

Refrigerate promptly; do not freeze.

NUTRIENT INFORMATION (serving size: 1¼ cups):
Calories: 230; Protein: 13.1 g; Carbohydrates: 42.2 g; Fat: 2.3 g; Fiber: 13.5 g

OTHER BENEFICIAL NUTRIENTS:
Excellent source of: vitamin A, vitamin C, folacin, fiber
Good source of: vitamin B_6, iron, zinc

black bean salsa

INGREDIENTS

1½ cups cooked black beans

½ cup frozen whole kernel corn, thawed

½ cup chopped onion

1 cup seeded and chopped tomato

1 fresh serrano pepper, seeded and chopped

1 Tbsp. balsamic vinegar

1 clove garlic, minced

1 tsp. NutriFit Calypso Salt Free Spice Blend

¼ cup chopped cilantro

DIRECTIONS

Note: For each teaspoon of the NutriFit Calypso Salt Free Spice Blend you may substitute: ½ tsp. ground chiles, ¼ tsp. cumin, ⅛ tsp. black pepper, and ⅛ tsp. garlic powder.

In a nonreactive bowl combine all the ingredients; mix well. Refrigerated, salsa will stay fresh for up to three days.

STORAGE INSTRUCTIONS

Refrigerate promptly; do not freeze.

NUTRIENT INFORMATION (serving size: ¼ cup):
Calories: 27; Protein: 1.5 g; Carbohydrates: 6.2 g; Fat: 0.1 g; Fiber: 1.7 g

OTHER BENEFICIAL NUTRIENTS:
Good source of: vitamin A

black bean, corn, and barley salad

SERVINGS: 4

INGREDIENTS

2¾ cups water

¾ cup medium pearled barley

2 cups cooked black beans

1 cup frozen peas, thawed

2 cups frozen corn, thawed

3 Tbsp. balsamic vinegar

2 Tbsp. minced basil

2 Tbsp. reduced-sodium
vegetable broth

1 Tbsp. canola oil

2 Tbsp. grated fat-free
Parmesan cheese

DIRECTIONS

1 In a 2-quart saucepan, bring the water and barley to a boil over high heat. Reduce the heat to medium-low; partially cover and simmer for 30–35 minutes, or until tender. Drain off any remaining water. Transfer the barley to a large bowl.

2 Add the beans, peas, and corn.

3 In a small bowl, whisk together the vinegar, basil, broth, and oil. Pour over the salad; toss to mix well. Sprinkle with the cheese. Serve warm or chilled.

STORAGE INSTRUCTIONS

Refrigerate promptly; do not freeze.

NUTRIENT INFORMATION (serving size: 2 cups):
Calories: 223; Protein: 9 g; Carbohydrates: 42 g; Fat: 3 g; Fiber: 9 g

OTHER BENEFICIAL NUTRIENTS:
Excellent source of: vitamin A, folacin, fiber
Good source of: iron

black-eyed pea and legume salad

SERVINGS: 6

INGREDIENTS

½ cup dried black-eyed peas

½ cup dried lentils

1 cup frozen green peas, thawed

1 cup carrots, cut into ⅛-inch-thick slices

½ cup finely chopped onion

¼ cup chopped parsley

1½ tsp. lemon juice

1 tsp. Dijon mustard

1 clove garlic, minced

1 tsp. NutriFit Lemon Garden Salt Free Spice Blend

1 tsp. olive oil

2 Tbsp. reduced-sodium vegetable broth

DIRECTIONS

Note: For each teaspoon of the NutriFit Lemon Garden Salt Free Spice Blend you may substitute: ¼ tsp. basil, ¼ tsp. marjoram, ¼ tsp. black pepper, and ¼ tsp. dill weed.

1 Place the black-eyed peas (rinsed and sorted) in a medium-size saucepan, with cold water to cover by 2 inches. Bring to a boil over medium heat; cover, reduce the heat to low, and simmer for 30 minutes. Add the lentils (rinsed and sorted) and cook until they are tender, adding more water if necessary.

2 Drain the peas and lentils, then transfer them to a medium-size bowl. Stir in the green peas, carrots, onion, and parsley.

3 For the dressing, mix the lemon juice, mustard, garlic, and spice blend together in a small bowl. Slowly whisk in the oil, then add the broth, whisking constantly. Pour the dressing over the peas and lentils and toss well.

STORAGE INSTRUCTIONS

Refrigerate promptly; may be frozen.

NUTRIENT INFORMATION (serving size: 1 cup):
Calories: 102; Protein: 7.3 g; Carbohydrates: 16.5 g; Fat: 1.2 g; Fiber: 8.1 g

OTHER BENEFICIAL NUTRIENTS:
Excellent source of: vitamin A, folacin, fiber
Good source of: iron

blueberry lemon coffee cake

SERVINGS: 9

INGREDIENTS

Canola oil cooking spray

1¾ cups white whole-wheat flour

¾ cup sugar

1¾ tsp. baking powder

¼ tsp. salt

2 tsp. grated lemon peel

1 cup fat-free evaporated milk

½ cup fat-free egg substitute

3 Tbsp. canola oil

1 cup blueberries

DIRECTIONS

1 Preheat the oven to 400°F. Coat a 9-inch square baking pan with canola oil spray.

2 In a medium bowl, mix the flour, sugar, baking powder, salt, and lemon peel with a spoon. Stir in the milk, egg substitute, and canola oil until blended.

3 Gently fold in the blueberries. Spread the batter in the prepared pan.

4 Bake for 20–25 minutes, or until golden brown. Cool for 10 minutes; remove from the pan and cool thoroughly, or serve warm.

STORAGE INSTRUCTIONS

Store at room temperature; may be frozen.

NUTRIENT INFORMATION (serving size: one 3-inch square):
Calories: 196; Protein: 4.9 g; Carbohydrates: 39.4 g; Fat: 2.1 g; Fiber: 1.1 g

OTHER BENEFICIAL NUTRIENTS:
Excellent source of: vitamin A
Good source of: vitamin C, calcium

blueberry whole-wheat pancakes

INGREDIENTS

¾ cup whole-wheat flour

¾ cup unbleached all-purpose flour

2 tsp. baking powder

4 tsp. sugar

¼ cup fat-free egg substitute

1¼ cups fat-free milk

1½ Tbsp. canola oil

¼ cup blueberries

Canola oil cooking spray

DIRECTIONS

1 In a small bowl, stir together the two flours, baking powder, and sugar; set aside.

2 In a large bowl, combine the egg substitute, milk, and oil. Add to the flour mixture and stir just until the dry ingredients are moistened (batter will be lumpy). Stir in the blueberries.

3 Lightly coat a 14-inch griddle with cooking spray and heat. For each pancake, spoon about 3 Tbsp. of the batter onto the griddle; spread to make a 4-inch circle. Cook for about 3 minutes, until the pancakes are bubbly on top; turn and cook for about 2 minutes more, until browned on the bottom.

STORAGE INSTRUCTIONS

Refrigerate promptly; may be frozen.

NUTRIENT INFORMATION (serving size: 4 pancakes):
Calories: 350; Protein: 12.9 g; Carbohydrates: 58 g; Fat: 7.9 g; Fiber: 4.9 g

OTHER BENEFICIAL NUTRIENTS:
Excellent source of: vitamin A, calcium, fiber
Good source of: folacin, iron, zinc

bran raisin muffins

SERVINGS: 8

INGREDIENTS

1½ cups unbleached
all-purpose flour

⅔ cup firmly packed brown
sugar

1 tsp. baking soda

½ tsp. cinnamon

¼ tsp. salt

¼ cup fat-free egg substitute

1½ cups fat-free milk

2 Tbsp. canola oil

3 cups unsweetened bran flakes
cereal

⅓ cup raisins

DIRECTIONS

1 Preheat the oven to 400°F. Line an 8-hole muffin tin
with paper or foil liners.

2 In a large bowl, mix the flour, sugar, baking soda, cinnamon, and salt. Beat the egg substitute in a small bowl
with the milk and oil. Add to the flour mixture, stirring
just until moistened (batter will be lumpy). Stir in the
cereal and raisins.

3 Spoon the batter into the prepared pan, filling each cup
two-thirds full. Bake for 20–25 minutes, or until lightly
browned. Serve warm.

STORAGE INSTRUCTIONS

Refrigerate promptly; may be frozen.

NUTRIENT INFORMATION (serving size: 1 muffin):
Calories: 181; Protein: 4 g; Carbohydrates: 36.9 g; Fat: 2.8 g; Fiber: 2.6 g

brown rice

SERVINGS: 3

INGREDIENTS

1 cup water

¼ tsp. salt

½ cup long-grain brown rice

DIRECTIONS

1 In a small saucepan, bring the water to a boil, covered, and add the salt. Then add the rice, stirring once.

2 Reduce the heat, cover, and simmer the rice for about 20 minutes. You can check the rice periodically and give it a stir to make certain that it doesn't burn.

STORAGE INSTRUCTIONS

Refrigerate promptly; may be frozen.

NUTRIENT INFORMATION (serving size: ½ cup):
Calories: 100; Protein: 2 g; Carbohydrates: 21.3 g; Fat: 0.7g; Fiber: 0.7 g

cheese omelet

SERVINGS: 1

INGREDIENTS

1½ cups fat-free egg substitute

¼ tsp. NutriFit Calypso Salt Free Spice Blend

Canola oil cooking spray

2 Tbsp. shredded reduced-fat cheddar cheese

DIRECTIONS

Note: For each teaspoon of the NutriFit Calypso Salt Free Spice Blend you may substitute: ½ tsp. ground chiles, ¼ tsp. cumin, ⅛ tsp. black pepper, and ⅛ tsp. garlic powder.

1 In a small bowl, whisk the egg substitute and spice blend together.

2 Heat a nonstick skillet, spray with cooking spray, and pour the egg mixture into the pan. Cook, allowing the eggs to set and lifting up the edges of the omelet as it forms to allow the liquid to run to the bottom of the skillet. This will allow the bottom of the omelet to cook. Turn when the eggs have set, and add the cheese on the bottom half of the omelet. Fold the top half over the cheese, forming a half-moon shape.

3 Serve immediately.

STORAGE INSTRUCTIONS

Refrigerate promptly; do not freeze.

NUTRIENT INFORMATION (serving size: 1 omelet):
Calories: 220; Protein: 40 g; Carbohydrates: 4 g; Fat: 3 g; Fiber: 0.5 g

OTHER BENEFICIAL NUTRIENTS:
Good source of: vitamin A

chicken fajitas

INGREDIENTS

1 lb. boneless, skinless chicken breasts, cut into ½-inch strips

1 Tbsp. NutriFit Calypso Salt Free Spice Blend

1 tsp. extra-virgin olive oil

2 cloves garlic, sliced

½ red onion, peeled and sliced

1 green bell pepper, cut into ¼-inch strips

1 yellow bell pepper, cut into ¼-inch strips

1 red bell pepper, cut into ¼-inch strips

⅔ cup fresh salsa, medium spicy

DIRECTIONS

Note: For each teaspoon of the NutriFit Calypso Salt Free Spice Blend you may substitute: ½ tsp. ground chiles, ¼ tsp. cumin, ⅛ tsp. black pepper, and ⅛ tsp. garlic powder.

1 Season the chicken with the spice blend. Cover the chicken with plastic wrap and marinate in the refrigerator for at least 30 minutes.

2 Heat a medium-size sauté pan, add the oil, garlic, onion, and bell peppers, and sauté over high heat for about 3 minutes.

3 Add the chicken and cook over high heat for 10 minutes, or until the meat is cooked, stirring constantly. Serve immediately with salsa on the side.

STORAGE INSTRUCTIONS

Refrigerate promptly; may be frozen.

NUTRIENT INFORMATION (serving size: 8 oz. mixture):
Calories: 298; Protein: 49 g; Carbohydrates: 11.2 g; Fat: 5.9 g; Fiber: 3.1 g

OTHER BENEFICIAL NUTRIENTS:
Excellent source of: vitamin A, vitamin C, vitamin B_6
Good source of: folacin, iron, zinc, fiber

chicken salad

SERVINGS: 4

INGREDIENTS

1 lb. boneless, skinless chicken breasts, cooked

1 tsp. NutriFit Mediterranean Salt Free Spice Blend

½ cup diced celery

3 whole green onions, chopped

½ cup fat-free mayonnaise

¼ tsp. paprika

DIRECTIONS

Note: For each teaspoon of the NutriFit Mediterranean Salt Free Spice Blend you may substitute: ¼ tsp. basil, ¼ tsp. oregano, ¼ tsp. garlic powder, and ¼ tsp. black pepper.

1 Cut the cooked chicken into cubes, and sprinkle with the spice blend.

2 Put the chicken in a bowl, then add the celery and onion. Combine the mayonnaise and paprika, then fold into the chicken mixture.

STORAGE INSTRUCTIONS

Refrigerate promptly; do not freeze.

NUTRIENT INFORMATION (serving size: ¾ cup):
Calories: 150; Protein: 26.5 g; Carbohydrates: 5.2 g; Fat: 1.5 g; Fiber: 0.5 g

OTHER BENEFICIAL NUTRIENTS:
Excellent source of: vitamin A, vitamin B_6

chicken salad with spiced sesame sauce

SERVINGS: 6

INGREDIENTS

3 (4-oz.) boneless, skinless chicken breasts

2 green onions, one trimmed and separated into white and green parts and the other chopped

1 slice fresh ginger

1 Tbsp. dry sherry

2 cups water, plus 1 Tbsp.

2 Tbsp. sesame tahini

2 Tbsp. reduced-sodium soy sauce

1½ tsp. distilled white vinegar

½ tsp. sesame oil

¼ tsp. cayenne pepper

1 Tbsp. chopped cilantro

3 cups shredded romaine lettuce

DIRECTIONS

1 In a 2-quart saucepan, combine the chicken, 1 whole green onion, the ginger, sherry, and 2 cups water. Bring to a boil over medium heat, cover, and simmer for about 20 minutes, until the meat in the thickest portion is no longer pink when cut. Remove the chicken from the broth and let stand just until cool enough to handle. Shred the chicken and set aside.

2 In a small bowl, combine the sesame tahini, soy sauce, and vinegar. Blend in the sesame oil, cayenne pepper, chopped green onion, and cilantro. Whisk until thoroughly blended. Mix in the remaining water.

3 To serve, mound the lettuce on a platter or individual plates. Arrange the chicken over the lettuce. Drizzle with the sesame sauce.

STORAGE INSTRUCTIONS

Refrigerate promptly; do not freeze.

NUTRIENT INFORMATION (serving size: ¾ cup):
Calories: 166; Protein: 27.1 g; Carbohydrates: 8.3 g; Fat: 1.6 g; Fiber: 1.4 g

OTHER BENEFICIAL NUTRIENTS:
Excellent source of: vitamin A, vitamin B_6
Good source of: vitamin C, folacin

chicken teriyaki

INGREDIENTS

1 lb. boneless, skinless chicken breasts

2 Tbsp. reduced-sodium teriyaki sauce marinade

Extra-virgin olive oil cooking spray

1 tsp. sesame seeds, toasted

DIRECTIONS

1 Wash the chicken and pat dry with paper towels. Marinate the chicken in the teriyaki marinade, covered and refrigerated, for at least 30 minutes, or up to one day.

2 Preheat the oven to 400°F. Coat a baking sheet with cooking spray.

3 Place the chicken on the prepared baking sheet and sprinkle with the sesame seeds. Bake for 10–15 minutes, or until the chicken tests done.

STORAGE INSTRUCTIONS

Refrigerate promptly; may be frozen.

NUTRIENT INFORMATION (serving size: 5 oz.):
Calories: 190; Protein: 36 g; Carbohydrates: 3.5 g; Fat: 2.4 g; Fiber: 0.1 g

OTHER BENEFICIAL NUTRIENTS:
Excellent source of: vitamin B_6
Good source of: vitamin A, iron, zinc

chicken with creamy herb sauce

SERVINGS: 4

INGREDIENTS

¾ cup water, plus 1 Tbsp.

¾ cup reduced-sodium chicken broth

¼ cup dry white wine

1 lb. boneless, skinless chicken breasts

½ tsp. cornstarch

6 oz. reduced-fat cream cheese with garlic and spices

2 Tbsp. chopped parsley (garnish)

DIRECTIONS

1 In a large skillet, bring ¾ cup water, the broth, and wine to a boil; add the chicken. Cover and reduce the heat. Simmer for 15 minutes. Remove the chicken from the skillet and set it aside to keep warm.

2 Bring the cooking liquid to a boil; cook for 5 minutes, or until reduced to ⅔ cup. Combine the remaining 1 Tbsp. water and cornstarch; add to the skillet. Bring to a boil and cook for 1 minute, stirring constantly. Add the cream cheese spread and cook until the mixture is thoroughly blended, stirring constantly.

3 Spoon the sauce over the chicken. Sprinkle with the parsley. Serve with brown rice.

STORAGE INSTRUCTIONS

Refrigerate promptly; may be frozen.

NUTRIENT INFORMATION (serving size: 5 oz. chicken breast / ½ cup rice):
Calories: 211; Protein: 39 g; Carbohydrates: 3.3 g; Fat: 2 g; Fiber: 0.7 g

OTHER BENEFICIAL NUTRIENTS:
Excellent source of: vitamin A, vitamin B$_6$

chilled apricot-pear soup

SERVINGS: 4

INGREDIENTS

1 (16 oz.) can pear halves in juice

1 (16 oz.) can apricot halves in juice

8 oz. plain fat-free yogurt

½ cup fat-free milk

1 tsp. NutriFit Certainly Cinnamon Salt Free Spice Blend

DIRECTIONS

Note: For each teaspoon of the NutriFit Certainly Cinnamon Salt Free Blend you may substitute: ½ tsp. cinnamon, ¼ tsp. nutmeg, ⅛ tsp. ginger, and ⅛ tsp. cloves.

1 Drain the canned fruit, reserving 1 cup of juice. Combine the canned fruit, reserved juice, yogurt, milk, and spice blend in a blender; cover and process for 1 minute or until smooth, stopping once to scrape down the sides of the container.

2 Cover and chill before serving.

STORAGE INSTRUCTIONS

Refrigerate promptly; do not freeze.

NUTRIENT INFORMATION (serving size: 1 cup):
Calories: 156; Protein: 5.4 g; Carbohydrates: 35.2 g; Fat: 0.2 g; Fiber: 3.8 g

OTHER BENEFICIAL NUTRIENTS:
Excellent source of: vitamin A, calcium
Good source of: vitamin C, fiber

chinese cabbage ramen salad

SERVINGS: 6

INGREDIENTS

⅓ cup seasoned rice vinegar

¼ cup reduced-sodium chicken broth

¼ cup pineapple juice

1 Tbsp. sugar or sugar equivalent

1 Tbsp. sesame oil

2 tsp. reduced-sodium soy sauce

2 Tbsp. sesame seeds, toasted (optional)

6 cups shredded green cabbage

1 pkg. reduced-fat ramen soup noodles, crumbled (discard the seasoning packet)

½ cup chopped cilantro

½ cup chopped green onions

DIRECTIONS

1 For the dressing, combine the vinegar, broth, juice, sugar, oil, and soy sauce in a small bowl; set aside.

2 Pour the sesame seeds (optional) into a small, dry skillet; toast until golden. In a large bowl, combine the sesame seeds, cabbage, uncooked noodles, cilantro, and green onions. Add the dressing and toss until the cabbage mixture is coated.

3 Cover and chill for at least 30 minutes, to allow time for the flavors to blend.

STORAGE INSTRUCTIONS

Refrigerate promptly; do not freeze.

BODY AFTER BABY

NUTRIENT INFORMATION (serving size: 2 cups):
Calories: 216; Protein: 5.4 g; Carbohydrates: 26.8 g; Fat: 10 g; Fiber: 3.4 g

OTHER BENEFICIAL NUTRIENTS:
Excellent source of: vitamin A, vitamin C, folacin
Good source of: fiber

chocolate chip fondue

SERVINGS: 12

INGREDIENTS

1 cup chocolate chips (you may use the reduced-fat variety)

¾ cup fat-free evaporated milk

1 (2.5-oz.) jar baby food prunes

Fresh fruit for dipping

DIRECTIONS

1 In a heavy saucepan, combine the chocolate chips and milk over low heat. Stir until smooth, making certain the mixture does not burn.

2 Add the prunes slowly, stirring constantly. If using as a fondue, keep warm in a fondue pot.

3 Fondue is great with all fruits, especially bananas, oranges, and pineapple, and is also good with small pieces of cake or graham crackers.

STORAGE INSTRUCTIONS

Refrigerate promptly; do not freeze.

NUTRIENT INFORMATION (serving size: 3 Tbsp.):
Calories: 125; Protein: 2.3 g; Carbohydrates: 23.4 g; Fat: 4.9 g; Fiber: 1.6 g

OTHER BENEFICIAL NUTRIENTS:
Excellent source of: vitamin A, vitamin C

chocolate chip spice cake

SERVINGS: 20

INGREDIENTS

Canola oil cooking spray

2 cups unbleached all-purpose flour

1 cup sugar

½ cup trans fat–free light margarine or spread

1 tsp. baking soda

1 tsp. cinnamon

½ tsp. ground cloves

1 cup reduced-fat buttermilk

⅓ cup mini chocolate chips

¼ cup fat-free egg substitute

DIRECTIONS

1 Preheat the oven to 375°F. Lightly spray a 9x13-inch sheet pan.

2 In a bowl, combine the flour, sugar, and margarine. Rub the mixture together with your hands, or cut in the margarine with a pastry blender, until the mixture is crumb-like. Add the baking soda, cinnamon, and cloves, mixing lightly.

3 Add the buttermilk, chocolate chips, and egg substitute. Gently stir the cake batter with a fork to incorporate the liquid. Do not overmix.

4 Pour the batter evenly into the prepared pan. Bake for about 20 minutes, until the cake springs back gently to the touch.

STORAGE INSTRUCTIONS

Store at room temperature; may be frozen.

NUTRIENT INFORMATION (serving size: one 2-inch square):
Calories: 125; Protein: 1.7 g; Carbohydrates: 22.1 g; Fat: 3.4 g; Fiber: 0.8 g

OTHER BENEFICIAL NUTRIENTS:
Excellent source of: vitamin A

chocolate pecan cake

SERVINGS: 12

INGREDIENTS

⅔ cup sugar

⅔ cup unbleached all-purpose flour

1 tsp. baking powder

Pinch salt

2 eggs

½ cup fat-free egg substitute

3½ oz. semisweet mini chocolate chips

4 Tbsp. trans fat–free light margarine or spread

1 tsp. vanilla extract

¼ cup chopped pecans

DIRECTIONS

1 Preheat the oven to 350°F. Coat a springform pan or tart tin with cooking spray and flour. Grind the sugar in a food processor or coffee grinder to make it superfine (optional). Sift the flour with the baking powder and salt to make self-rising flour. Set aside.

2 Beat the eggs and egg substitute until very thick and light yellow. Add the reserved sugar and continue beating. Meanwhile, melt the chocolate and margarine in the microwave. Stir until the mixture is smooth. Add the chocolate mixture to the egg mixture and continue beating until slightly thickened.

3 Gently fold in the flour, vanilla, and pecans. Pour into the prepared pan.

4 Bake for 20 minutes, or until a toothpick inserted in the center comes out clean. Turn off the oven and let cool in the oven for 10 minutes.

STORAGE INSTRUCTIONS

Store at room temperature; may be frozen.

NUTRIENT INFORMATION (serving size: one 2-inch wedge):
Calories: 214; Protein: 3.7 g; Carbohydrates: 39.7 g; Fat: 5 g; Fiber: 0.7 g

OTHER BENEFICIAL NUTRIENTS:
Excellent source of: vitamin A

chocolate tofu pudding

INGREDIENTS

1 large ripe banana, peeled

⅓ cup honey

1 Tbsp. canola oil

1 (12.3-oz.) pkg. extra-firm, reduced-fat tofu, drained

3 Tbsp. water

2 Tbsp. unsweetened cocoa powder

1 Tbsp. unsweetened applesauce

¼ tsp. vanilla extract

¼ tsp. chocolate extract (optional)

DIRECTIONS

1 In a food processor or blender, combine the banana, honey, and oil. Add the tofu piece by piece, blending after each addition. If the mixture is too thick (which will depend on the amount of moisture in your tofu), add water 1 tablespoon at a time, until the mixture reaches a pudding consistency.

2 Add the cocoa, applesauce, and the extracts, and process or blend until smooth. Serve immediately.

STORAGE INSTRUCTIONS

Refrigerate promptly; do not freeze.

NUTRIENT INFORMATION (serving size: ½ cup):
Calories: 370; Protein: 14 g; Carbohydrates: 64 g; Fat: 8 g; Fiber: 1.6 g

OTHER BENEFICIAL NUTRIENTS:
Excellent source of: vitamin A, vitamin B_6
Good source of: vitamin C, calcium, iron

chunky mashed yams

SERVINGS: 1

INGREDIENTS

½ cup yams or sweet potatoes, peeled and cut into ½-inch dice

1 cup reduced-sodium vegetable broth

½ tsp. trans fat–free light margarine or spread

⅛ tsp. white pepper

DIRECTIONS

1 In a small covered saucepan, cook the yams in the vegetable broth for about 15 minutes, until soft.

2 Drain off the excess broth, leaving the yams very moist. Add the margarine and pepper and mash gently with a fork, just until a desired texture is reached.

STORAGE INSTRUCTIONS

Refrigerate promptly; do not freeze.

NUTRIENT INFORMATION (serving size: 1 cup):
Calories: 233; Protein: 3.9 g; Carbohydrates: 55.1 g; Fat: 0.3 g; Fiber: 6.9 g

OTHER BENEFICIAL NUTRIENTS:
Excellent source of: vitamin A, vitamin C, vitamin B_6, folacin, fiber

cinnamon french toast

INGREDIENTS

½ cup fat-free egg substitute

½ cup 1 percent milk

1 tsp. cinnamon

1 tsp. vanilla extract

6 slices whole-wheat cinnamon bread

Canola oil cooking spray

DIRECTIONS

1 In a bowl, mix together the egg substitute, milk, cinnamon, and vanilla.

2 Pour the mixture into a baking dish large enough to hold the bread slices in a single layer. Dip the bread into the batter, coating the slices well.

3 Heat a griddle or skillet, then spray with cooking spray, and put the slices on the hot griddle. Cook until golden, then turn and cook the other side until thoroughly cooked. Serve immediately.

STORAGE INSTRUCTIONS

Refrigerate promptly; may be frozen.

NUTRIENT INFORMATION (serving size: 1 slice):
Calories: 129; Protein: 5 g; Carbohydrates: 20.7 g; Fat: 2.6 g; Fiber: 1.1 g

OTHER BENEFICIAL NUTRIENTS:
Excellent source of: vitamin A
Good source of: folacin

cinnamon spread

SERVINGS: 16

INGREDIENTS

1 cup fat-free cottage cheese

2 Tbsp. frozen apple-juice concentrate

1 tsp. grated lemon peel

1 tsp. lemon juice

1 cup fat-free sour cream

¼ tsp. NutriFit Certainly Cinnamon Salt Free Spice Blend

DIRECTIONS

Note: For each teaspoon of the NutriFit Certainly Cinnamon Salt Free Spice Blend you may substitute: ½ tsp. cinnamon, ¼ tsp. nutmeg, ⅛ tsp. ginger, and ⅛ tsp. cloves.

1 In a food processor or blender, process the cottage cheese until all of the curds disappear and the mixture is creamy. Add the apple-juice concentrate, lemon peel, and lemon juice and process until well blended.

2 Empty the mixture into a bowl, stir in the sour cream and spice blend, and store, covered, in the refrigerator. Will keep for 3-4 weeks if fresh ingredients are used.

STORAGE INSTRUCTIONS

Refrigerate promptly; do not freeze.

NUTRIENT INFORMATION (serving size: 2 Tbsp.):
Calories: 15; Protein: 1.4 g; Carbohydrates: 2 g; Fat: 0 g; Fiber: 0 g

OTHER BENEFICIAL NUTRIENTS:
Good source of: vitamin A

cocoa fruit nougats

INGREDIENTS

1¼ cups dried figs

2½ cups mixed dried fruits, such as apples, apricots, pears, and prunes

½ cup unsweetened cocoa powder

2 Tbsp. orange juice

2 Tbsp. honey

DIRECTIONS

1 Remove the stems from the figs and the pits from the prunes, if necessary. Using the metal blade of a food processor, process the dried fruits and figs until ground and almost paste-like.

2 In a large bowl, combine the cocoa, orange juice, and honey with the fruit mixture; mix well. Cover and refrigerate until chilled.

3 Shape the mixture into 1¼-inch balls. Store in an airtight container in the refrigerator.

STORAGE INSTRUCTIONS

Refrigerate promptly; do not freeze.

NUTRIENT INFORMATION (serving size: 2 balls):
Calories: 51; Protein: 0.6 g; Carbohydrates: 13.2 g; Fat: 0.1 g; Fiber: 1.4 g

OTHER BENEFICIAL NUTRIENTS:
Excellent source of: vitamin A

COUSCOUS

SERVINGS: 2

INGREDIENTS

¾ cup reduced-sodium chicken broth

½ cup uncooked whole-wheat couscous

1 tsp. finely chopped parsley

DIRECTIONS

1 In a saucepan, bring the broth to a boil. Remove from the heat. Add the couscous.

2 Cover and let stand for 2–3 minutes, or until the couscous has absorbed the liquid.

3 Fluff the couscous with a fork. Sprinkle with parsley and serve.

STORAGE INSTRUCTIONS

Refrigerate promptly; may be frozen.

NUTRIENT INFORMATION (serving size: ½ cup):
Calories: 226; Protein: 9.1 g; Carbohydrates: 46 g; Fat: 0.5 g; Fiber: 7 g

OTHER BENEFICIAL NUTRIENTS:
Excellent source of: fiber
Good source of: iron

couscous-stuffed squash

SERVINGS: 2

INGREDIENTS

1 large acorn squash

2 tsp. NutriFit Lemon Garden Salt Free Spice Blend

1 tsp. olive oil

1 large zucchini, coarsely chopped

½ cup chopped green onions

2 cloves garlic, minced

1 cup reduced-sodium V8 juice

1 cup uncooked whole-wheat couscous

3 oz. reduced-fat feta cheese, crumbled

DIRECTIONS

Note: For each teaspoon of the NutriFit Lemon Garden Salt Free Spice Blend you may substitute: ¼ tsp. basil, ¼ tsp. marjoram, ¼ tsp. black pepper, and ¼ tsp. dill weed.

1 Wash the squash and cut it in half. Spoon out and discard the seeds. Season both sides with some of the spice blend and place in a microwave-safe glass dish, flesh side down. Cover with plastic wrap and cook on High for 10 minutes, or until the flesh is tender. Cool slightly, and a scoop the flesh out with a spoon; set aside. Reserve the shells.

2 Preheat the oven to 350°F.

3 Heat a large nonstick skillet and add the oil. Then add the zucchini, green onions, garlic, and remaining spice blend. Cook for 4–6 minutes, or until the vegetables are tender, stirring often. Stir in the juice and bring to a boil. Stir in the couscous; cover. Remove from the heat and let stand for 5 minutes, or until the couscous is soft. Fluff with a fork.

4 Add the couscous mixture and the feta cheese to the squash. Toss to mix well. Divide between the reserved squash shells. Cover each shell with foil, place in a 9x13-inch baking dish, and bake for 15–20 minutes, or until heated through.

STORAGE INSTRUCTIONS

Refrigerate promptly; do not freeze.

NUTRIENT INFORMATION (serving size: ½ squash):
Calories: 290; Protein: 13 g; Carbohydrates: 47.8 g; Fat: 5.6 g; Fiber: 8.3 g

OTHER BENEFICIAL NUTRIENTS:
Excellent source of: vitamin A, vitamin C, fiber
Good source of: calcium

couscous with raisins and dates

INGREDIENTS

¾ cup unsweetened apple juice

¾ cup water

1 cup uncooked couscous

2 Tbsp. raisins

2 Tbsp. diced unsweetened dates

¼ tsp. NutriFit Certainly Cinnamon Salt Free Spice Blend

DIRECTIONS

Note: For each teaspoon of the NutriFit Certainly Cinnamon Salt Free Spice Blend you may substitute: ½ tsp. cinnamon, ¼ tsp. nutmeg, ⅛ tsp. ginger, and ⅛ tsp. cloves.

1 In a medium saucepan, combine the juice and water and bring to a boil. Remove from the heat. Add the couscous, raisins, dates, and spice blend; cover and let stand for 5 minutes, or until the couscous is tender and the liquid is absorbed.

2 Fluff the couscous with a fork, and transfer it to a large serving bowl. Add more juice before serving, if needed.

STORAGE INSTRUCTIONS

Refrigerate promptly; do not freeze.

NUTRIENT INFORMATION (serving size: ½ cup):
Calories: 114; Protein: 3.1 g; Carbohydrates: 24.8 g; Fat: 0.2 g; Fiber: 1.5 g

creamy herb dressing

INGREDIENTS

½ cup fat-free sour cream

⅓ cup fat-free mayonnaise

½ cup 1 percent milk

1 tsp. thyme

⅛ tsp. ground white pepper

3 Tbsp. chopped green onions

2 tsp. finely chopped Italian parsley

2 tsp. chopped dill

2 tsp. chopped basil

2 tsp. grated fat-free Parmesan cheese

DIRECTIONS

1 In a food processor or blender, combine the sour cream, mayonnaise, and milk. Process until thoroughly combined, scraping down the sides of the container as necessary.

2 Stir in the remaining ingredients. Transfer the mixture to a bowl or jar with a tight-fitting lid. Cover and refrigerate until ready to use. Stir well before serving. Refrigerated, this dressing will remain fresh for about one week.

STORAGE INSTRUCTIONS

Refrigerate promptly; do not freeze.

BODY AFTER BABY

NUTRIENT INFORMATION (serving size: ¼ cup):
Calories: 46; Protein: 2.2 g; Carbohydrates: 7 g; Fat: 0.2 g; Fiber: 0.1 g

OTHER BENEFICIAL NUTRIENTS:
Excellent source of: vitamin A

crispy baked cod

SERVINGS: 4

INGREDIENTS

Canola oil cooking spray

1½ lbs. (4 medium fillets) cod

3 Tbsp. sesame seeds

¼ cup fat-free egg substitute

1 Tbsp. fat-free milk

1 Tbsp. lemon juice

1 tsp. Worcestershire sauce

½ cup cornmeal

1 tsp. NutriFit Calypso Salt Free Spice Blend

1 clove garlic, minced

DIRECTIONS

Note: For each teaspoon of the NutriFit Calypso Salt Free Spice Blend you may substitute: ½ tsp. ground chiles, ¼ tsp. cumin, ⅛ tsp. black pepper, and ⅛ tsp. garlic powder.

1 Preheat the oven to 425°F. Line a baking sheet with foil or baking parchment. Lightly spray it with cooking spray. Wash the fish, pat it dry, and place it on the prepared baking sheet.

2 To toast the sesame seeds, place in a dry, nonstick skillet over medium heat, stirring constantly, until fragrant and golden brown; set aside.

3 In a small bowl, combine the egg substitute, milk, lemon juice, and Worcestershire sauce. Using a pastry brush, brush the egg mixture onto the fillets. Mix together the cornmeal, spice blend, garlic, and sesame seeds. Sprinkle the cornmeal mixture over the fillets, coating them well. Lightly coat the coated fillets with cooking spray.

4 Bake for 10 minutes per inch of thickness, about 15 minutes. Serve immediately.

STORAGE INSTRUCTIONS

Best eaten within two days; do not freeze.

NUTRIENT INFORMATION (serving size: 1 fillet):
Calories: 248; Protein: 33.8 g; Carbohydrates: 16.2 g; Fat: 4.8 g; Fiber: 2.2 g

OTHER BENEFICIAL NUTRIENTS:
Excellent source of: vitamin A, vitamin B_6
Good source of: vitamin C, folacin, calcium, iron, zinc

dessert nachos

INGREDIENTS

Canola oil cooking spray

⅓ cup sugar

1 tsp. cinnamon

8 (10-inch) fat-free flour tortillas

2 cups diced strawberries

1 cup diced pineapple

2 cups diced cantaloupe

4 oz. Neufchâtel light cream cheese

4 oz. fat-free cream cheese

½ cup orange juice

3 Tbsp. honey

DIRECTIONS

1 Preheat the oven to 500°F. Lightly coat a baking sheet with cooking spray.

2 In a shallow bowl, mix the sugar and cinnamon; set aside. Dip the tortillas one at a time in water; let drain briefly. Stack the tortillas and cut into 6 or 8 wedges.

3 Dip one side of each wedge in the sugar mixture. Arrange the wedges in a single layer, sugar side up, on the prepared baking sheet.

4 Bake for 4–5 minutes, until crisp and golden. Let the chips cool, then store in an airtight container for up to three days.

5 Combine the fruit to make a salsa. You may vary the fruit as desired.

6 In a small saucepan, combine the Neufchâtel cheese, cream cheese, orange juice, and honey. Whisk over low heat for about 3 minutes, until the sauce is smooth.

7 Mound the chips on a platter. Offer the sauce and salsa to spoon over the chips.

STORAGE INSTRUCTIONS

Refrigerate promptly; do not freeze.

NUTRIENT INFORMATION (serving size: 6 wedges):
Calories: 206; Protein: 6.2 g; Carbohydrates: 38.9 g; Fat: 3.4 g; Fiber: 7.6 g

OTHER BENEFICIAL NUTRIENTS:
Excellent source of: vitamin A, vitamin C, fiber
Good source of: folacin, calcium

egg salad

INGREDIENTS

1 hard-boiled egg

1 Tbsp. diced celery

1 Tbsp. diced carrot

1 tsp. fat-free mayonnaise

⅛ tsp. NutriFit Lemon Garden
Salt Free Spice Blend

DIRECTIONS

Note: For each teaspoon of the NutriFit Lemon Garden Salt Free Spice Blend you may substitute: ¼ tsp. basil, ¼ tsp. marjoram, ¼ tsp. black pepper, and ¼ tsp. dill weed.

1 Chop the hard-boiled egg into small pieces.

2 In a small bowl, combine the egg, celery, carrot, mayonnaise, and spice blend.

3 Stir well until the mixture is blended.

STORAGE INSTRUCTIONS

Refrigerate promptly; do not freeze.

NUTRIENT INFORMATION (serving size: 1 salad):
Calories: 82; Protein: 6.4 g; Carbohydrates: 2.3 g; Fat: 5 g; Fiber: 0.3 g

OTHER BENEFICIAL NUTRIENTS:
Excellent source of: vitamin A
Good source of: folacin

eggless egg salad

SERVINGS: 3

INGREDIENTS

1 (12.3 oz.) pkg. extra-firm, reduced-fat tofu, drained

½ cup fat-free mayonnaise

2 tsp. mustard

1 tsp. apple-cider vinegar

1 tsp. honey

1 tsp. ground turmeric

2 Tbsp. diced celery

2 Tbsp. diced onion

1 tsp. chopped parsley

1 tsp. NutriFit Lemon Garden Salt Free Spice Blend

DIRECTIONS

Note: For each teaspoon of the NutriFit Lemon Garden Salt Free Spice Blend you may substitute: ¼ tsp. basil, ¼ tsp. marjoram, ¼ tsp. black pepper, and ¼ tsp. dill weed.

1 Drain the tofu and crumble it into a small bowl. Add the mayonnaise and mix well.

2 In a separate bowl, combine the mustard, vinegar, honey, and turmeric. Mix thoroughly and pour over the crumbled tofu. Add the celery, onion, parsley, and spice blend; mix thoroughly.

3 Cover and chill for at least 30 minutes, to allow time for the flavors to blend. It will stay fresh for up to two days.

STORAGE INSTRUCTIONS

Best eaten within two days; do not freeze.

NUTRIENT INFORMATION (serving size: 1 cup):
Calories: 83; Protein: 8.5 g; Carbohydrates: 7.7 g; Fat: 0.9 g; Fiber: 0.2 g

eggplant parmigiana

SERVINGS: 6

INGREDIENTS

3 lbs. eggplant, unpeeled

Extra-virgin olive oil cooking spray

1 Tbsp. NutriFit Mediterranean Salt Free Spice Blend

2 cups fat-free marinara sauce

1 cup reduced-fat, reduced-sodium ricotta cheese

1½ cups shredded reduced-fat mozzarella cheese

¼ cup grated fat-free Parmesan cheese

DIRECTIONS

Note: For each tablespoon of the NutriFit Mediterranean Salt Free Spice Blend you may substitute: 1 tsp. oregano, 1 tsp. basil, ½ tsp. black pepper, and ½ tsp. garlic powder.

1 Preheat the oven to 375°F.

2 Wash and slice the eggplants into ½-inch rounds. Line a baking sheet with parchment paper or foil, coat lightly with cooking spray, and spread the slices in a single layer (they may slightly overlap). Sprinkle with the spice blend. Bake until lightly browned, turn over, and repeat with the spray and spice blend. Bake until soft.

3 Lightly coat a 9x13-inch baking dish with cooking spray. Spoon a small amount of marinara sauce onto the bottom of the dish, then layer the eggplant slices over the sauce, crowding slightly to cover the surface of the dish. With a teaspoon, spread a small amount of the ricotta over each slice, then sprinkle each layer with a little mozzarella. Top with the Parmesan cheese, then repeat with layers of eggplant, ricotta, marinara sauce, mozzarella, and Parmesan until all of the ingredients are used up, ending with Parmesan cheese.

4 Bake for 30–45 minutes, or until the cheese is melted and the casserole is thoroughly heated.

STORAGE INSTRUCTIONS

Refrigerate promptly; may be frozen.

NUTRIENT INFORMATION
(serving size: 4-inch wedge):
Calories: 253; Protein: 30.3 g; Carbohydrates: 23.5 g; Fat: 5.1 g; Fiber: 6.7 g

OTHER BENEFICIAL NUTRIENTS:
Excellent source of: vitamin A, folacin, calcium, fiber
Good source of: vitamin C, vitamin B_6, iron, zinc

fish with sherry mushroom sauce

SERVINGS: 4

INGREDIENTS

2 Tbsp. olive oil

1 cup thinly sliced mushrooms

½ cup sliced green onion

1½ lb. cod or sea bass (4 fillets) (¾ inch thick)

Dash each salt and pepper

1 tsp. cornstarch

⅓ cup water

¼ cup dry sherry

1 Tbsp. reduced-sodium soy sauce

2 tsp. peeled and minced fresh ginger

Lemon wedges (for garnish)

DIRECTIONS

1 Heat a large skillet over medium-high heat. Add 1½ Tbsp. of the oil. Add the mushrooms and onions and cook, stirring, for about 5 minutes, until lightly browned. Remove from the pan; set aside.

2 Rinse the fish and pat dry. Heat the skillet again and add the remaining ½ Tbsp. of oil. Add the fish in a single layer. Season to taste with salt and pepper. Cover and cook for about 8 minutes, until just slightly translucent or wet inside when cut in the thickest part. With a wide spatula, lift out the fish and transfer to a warm platter; keep warm.

3 In a small cup or bowl, stir together the cornstarch, water, sherry, soy sauce, and ginger. Pour the mixture into the skillet; add the mushroom mixture and stir to loosen any browned bits. Cook over high heat, stirring, until the mixture comes to a boil and thickens and bubbles slightly, then pour the mixture over the fish.

4 Serve with lemon wedges for garnish.

STORAGE INSTRUCTIONS

Refrigerate until serving time; do not freeze.

NUTRIENT INFORMATION (serving size: one 6-oz. fillet):
Calories: 246; Protein: 31.7 g; Carbohydrates: 6.5 g; Fat: 8 g; Fiber: 1.3 g

OTHER BENEFICIAL NUTRIENTS:
Excellent source of: vitamin A, vitamin B_6, folacin
Good source of: vitamin C, iron

fragrant brown rice and peas

SERVINGS: 5

INGREDIENTS

1 cup uncooked brown rice

2 cups water

½ tsp. salt

1 cup frozen peas

DIRECTIONS

1 Place the rice in a colander and rinse it under running water for about 1 minute, until the water runs clear.

2 Bring the water to a boil in a 3-quart saucepan. Add the salt, stir in the rice, and cover the pan. Cook the rice over low heat for about 15 minutes, until tender and the liquid is absorbed.

3 Stir in the peas and let the rice stand for 10 minutes. Fluff with a fork before serving.

STORAGE INSTRUCTIONS

Refrigerate promptly; may be frozen.

NUTRIENT INFORMATION (serving size: ¾ cup):
Calories: 161; Protein: 4 g; Carbohydrates: 35 g; Fat: 0.1 g; Fiber: 2.6 g

OTHER BENEFICIAL NUTRIENTS:
Excellent source of: vitamin A
Good source of: folacin, fiber

fragrant kale

INGREDIENTS

¼ tsp. olive oil

1 Tbsp. finely chopped onion

2 cups finely sliced kale

⅛ tsp. NutriFit Calypso
Salt Free Spice Blend

DIRECTIONS

Note: For each teaspoon of the NutriFit Calypso Salt Free Spice Blend you may substitute: ½ tsp. ground chiles, ¼ tsp. cumin, ⅛ tsp. black pepper, and ⅛ tsp. garlic powder.

1 Heat a nonstick skillet. Add the oil and onions and sauté until softened.

2 Add the kale and spice blend and cook until wilted.

STORAGE INSTRUCTIONS

Refrigerate promptly; do not freeze.

NUTRIENT INFORMATION (serving size: 1 cup):
Calories: 55; Protein: 2.6 g; Carbohydrates: 8.2 g; Fat: 1.7 g; Fiber: 2.8 g

OTHER BENEFICIAL NUTRIENTS:
Excellent source of: vitamin A, vitamin C
Good source of: vitamin B_6, folacin, calcium, fiber

fragrant lentil soup

INGREDIENTS

6 cups reduced-sodium chicken broth

1½ cups uncooked red lentils, rinsed and drained

¼ cup grated onion

¼ tsp. ground cumin

½ cup water

1 tsp. NutriFit Lemon Garden Salt Free Spice Blend

⅛ tsp. cayenne pepper

1 Tbsp. chopped parsley

DIRECTIONS

Note: For each teaspoon of the NutriFit Lemon Garden Salt Free Spice Blend you may substitute: ¼ tsp. basil, ¼ tsp. marjoram, ¼ tsp. black pepper, and ¼ tsp. dill weed.

1 In a medium-size saucepan over medium heat, combine the broth, lentils, onion, cumin, water, spice blend, and cayenne pepper; partially cover and simmer for about 30 minutes, until lentils are soft.

2 Pour the mixture into a blender or a food processor and process until smooth (you may have to do this in batches).

3 Return the soup to the pan and simmer until it is the desired thickness, stirring frequently. Garnish with parsley.

STORAGE INSTRUCTIONS

Refrigerate promptly; may be frozen.

NUTRIENT INFORMATION (serving size: 2 cups):
Calories: 428; Protein: 21 g; Carbohydrates: 100.6 g; Fat: 2.4 g; Fiber: 28.7 g

OTHER BENEFICIAL NUTRIENTS:
Excellent source of: vitamin A, vitamin C, folacin, fiber
Good source of: vitamin B$_6$, calcium, iron, zinc

fresh baked rainbow trout

SERVINGS: 4

INGREDIENTS

1 tsp. olive oil

1 Tbsp. dry white wine

1 Tbsp. white-wine Worcestershire sauce

1 Tbsp. lemon juice

1 clove garlic, minced or pressed

1½ lbs. trout (4 fillets), cleaned

Extra-virgin olive oil cooking spray

DIRECTIONS

1 Preheat the oven to 350°F.

2 For the marinade, whisk the oil, wine, Worcestershire sauce, and lemon juice in a small bowl; stir in the garlic. Pour the marinade into a 13x9-inch glass baking dish.

3 Rinse the fish and pat it dry with paper towels. Place the fish in the baking dish; spoon the marinade over the fish to coat thoroughly. Marinate, covered, in the refrigerator for 30 minutes, turning the fish over occasionally.

4 Coat a baking dish with cooking spray. Arrange the trout in the baking dish, cover with foil, and bake for 15 minutes, or until the fish flakes easily.

STORAGE INSTRUCTIONS

Best eaten within two days; do not freeze.

BODY AFTER BABY

NUTRIENT INFORMATION (serving size: 6 oz.):
Calories: 236; Protein: 35.6 g; Carbohydrates: 5.8 g; Fat: 6.9 g; Fiber: 0.2 g

OTHER BENEFICIAL NUTRIENTS:
Excellent source of: vitamin A, vitamin B_6
Good source of: vitamin C, calcium, iron, zinc

fresh herb risotto with peas

SERVINGS: 4

INGREDIENTS

1 tsp. extra-virgin olive oil

½ cup chopped onion

½ cup chopped fennel

¾ cup uncooked short-grain brown rice

3 cups reduced-sodium vegetable broth

½ cup white wine

¼ cup dealcoholized white wine

¼ cup grated fat-free Parmesan cheese

1 cup frozen green peas, thawed

1 Tbsp. chopped Italian parsley

1 Tbsp. chopped basil

DIRECTIONS

1 Heat a large saucepan over medium-high heat, add the oil and sauté the onion for 3 minutes.

2 Add the fennel and rice and cook for 2 minutes, stirring until the rice is well coated.

3 Add 1 cup of the vegetable broth and the wine, and bring to a rolling boil, stirring until the liquid is absorbed.

4 Add another cup of the vegetable broth, bring back to a boil, and cook and stir until the broth is absorbed; repeat with one more cup of broth. This process should take about 25 minutes.

5 Stir in the cheese, peas, parsley, and basil.

STORAGE INSTRUCTIONS

Refrigerate promptly; may be frozen.

NUTRIENT INFORMATION (serving size: ⅔ cup):
Calories: 251; Protein: 7.6 g; Carbohydrates: 44.4 g; Fat: 1.3 g; Fiber: 3.7 g

OTHER BENEFICIAL NUTRIENTS:
Excellent source of: vitamin A
Good source of: vitamin C, folacin, fiber

fresh seasonal fruit salad

SERVINGS: 4

INGREDIENTS

⅔ cup cubed watermelon

½ cup seedless grapes

⅔ cup diced pineapple

⅔ cup orange sections, peeled and diced

⅔ cup cubed honeydew

⅔ cup cubed cantaloupe

DIRECTIONS

In a large bowl, combine all of the cut fruit. Cover and refrigerate. Serve chilled.

STORAGE INSTRUCTIONS

Refrigerate promptly; do not freeze.

NUTRIENT INFORMATION (serving size: 1 cup):
Calories: 65; Protein: 1.2 g; Carbohydrates: 16 g; Fat: 0.4 g; Fiber: 3.4 g

OTHER BENEFICIAL NUTRIENTS:
Excellent source of: vitamin A, vitamin C
Good source of: fiber

fresh spinach omelet

SERVINGS: 1

INGREDIENTS

1 cup fat-free egg substitute

1 dash NutriFit Calypso
Salt Free Spice Blend

1 cup fresh spinach, well
washed and ribs removed

Canola oil cooking spray

DIRECTIONS

Note: For each teaspoon of the NutriFit Calypso Salt Free Spice Blend
you may substitute: ½ tsp. ground chiles, ¼ tsp. cumin, ⅛ tsp. black
pepper, and ⅛ tsp. garlic powder.

1 In a small bowl, whisk the egg substitute and spice blend
   together.

2 Coat a nonstick skillet with the cooking spray and pour
   the egg mixture in the pan. Heat through on one side,
   add the spinach, fold the omelet, and turn it over, to
   complete cooking on the other side.

STORAGE INSTRUCTIONS

Best eaten within two days; do not freeze.

NUTRIENT INFORMATION (serving size: 1 omelet):
Calories: 132; Protein: 25.6 g; Carbohydrates: 4.8 g; Fat: 0.2 g; Fiber: 1.5 g

OTHER BENEFICIAL NUTRIENTS:
Excellent source of: vitamin A, vitamin C, folacin
Good source of: iron

fresh tomato salad

INGREDIENTS

4 cups romaine lettuce leaves

9 ripe tomatoes, cored and sliced (about 2 cups)

2 Tbsp. vegetable broth

1 Tbsp. balsamic vinegar

¼ cup finely chopped Italian parsley

½ tsp. finely chopped mint

1 Tbsp. olive oil

DIRECTIONS

1 Wash the lettuce leaves and pat them dry with paper towels. Arrange the lettuce leaves on four salad plates. Top the salad with the tomato slices.

2 In a small bowl, combine the broth, vinegar, and herbs. Whisk in the olive oil. Drizzle over the salads.

STORAGE INSTRUCTIONS

Refrigerate promptly; do not freeze.

NUTRIENT INFORMATION (serving size: 1½ cups):
Calories: 69; Protein: 2.3 g; Carbohydrates: 10.3 g; Fat: 3 g; Fiber: 2.7 g

OTHER BENEFICIAL NUTRIENTS:
Excellent source of: vitamin A, vitamin C, folacin
Good source of: fiber

fried rice with soybeans

INGREDIENTS

Canola oil cooking spray

½ cup fat-free egg substitute

1 tsp. canola oil

1½ cups fresh bean sprouts

⅓ cup shredded carrot

¼ cup thinly sliced green onion

2 cloves garlic, minced

1 tsp. sesame oil

4 cups cooked brown rice, cooled

1 Tbsp. reduced-sodium soy sauce

1 tsp. peeled and minced fresh ginger

1 lb. frozen edamame, shelled (soybeans)

DIRECTIONS

1 Heat a large nonstick rectangular griddle until hot. Spray with cooking spray and add the egg substitute. Cook for 2 minutes, or until set. Remove from the pan and dice the mixture. Keep warm.

2 Heat in a skillet over medium-high heat. Add the canola oil, sprouts, carrots, onions, and garlic; stir-fry for 1 minute.

3 Add the sesame oil, cooked rice, and the remaining ingredients. Stir-fry for 5 minutes, or until heated through.

STORAGE INSTRUCTIONS

Refrigerate promptly; may be frozen.

NUTRIENT INFORMATION (serving size: ¾ cup):
Calories: 229; Protein: 12.8 g; Carbohydrates: 30.5 g; Fat: 7.1 g; Fiber: 5.7 g

OTHER BENEFICIAL NUTRIENTS:
Excellent source of: vitamin A, folacin, fiber
Good source of: vitamin B_6, iron, zinc

fruit-and-nut granola

SERVINGS: 12

INGREDIENTS

¼ cup raw sunflower seeds

¼ cup sliced almonds

¼ cup raisins

2 cups oat flakes

1 cup Grape-Nuts cereal

¼ cup chopped dried pineapple

¼ cup chopped dried dates

¼ cup dried cranberries

1 cup bran flakes

1 cup apple chips (baked, not fried), broken up

DIRECTIONS

1 Preheat the oven to 350°F.

2 Place the sunflower seeds and almonds in a single layer on a baking sheet. Roast for 15 minutes.

3 In a large bowl, combine all the ingredients and store in an airtight container.

STORAGE INSTRUCTIONS

Store in a cool, dry place.

BODY AFTER BABY

NUTRIENT INFORMATION (serving size: ½ cup):
Calories: 172; Protein: 4.5 g; Carbohydrates: 34.1 g; Fat: 3.3 g; Fiber: 3.5 g

OTHER BENEFICIAL NUTRIENTS:
Excellent source of: vitamin A
Good source of: folacin, fiber

garbanzo pita pockets

SERVINGS: 4

INGREDIENTS

1 (15-oz.) can reduced-sodium garbanzo beans, drained and rinsed

1 small red bell pepper, diced

1 small green bell pepper, diced

1 small red onion, thinly sliced

1 clove garlic, minced

1 Tbsp. sliced black olives

1 Tbsp. sliced green olives

1 (6-oz.) jar marinated artichoke hearts, quartered, liquid reserved

2 Tbsp. red-wine vinegar

1 tsp. NutriFit Lemon Garden Salt Free Spice Blend

4 large pita breads

2 cups shredded romaine lettuce

DIRECTIONS

Note: For each teaspoon of the NutriFit Lemon Garden Salt Free Spice Blend you may substitute: ¼ tsp. basil, ¼ tsp. marjoram, ¼ tsp. black pepper, and ¼ tsp. dill weed.

1 In a large bowl, combine the garbanzo beans, peppers, onion, garlic, olives, artichokes and their liquid, vinegar, and spice blend; set aside.

2 Slice off the top third of each pita bread; open the bread to form a pocket. Place an equal amount of lettuce in each pita and fill with the garbanzo filling.

STORAGE INSTRUCTIONS

Refrigerate promptly; do not freeze.

NUTRIENT INFORMATION (serving size: 1 pita):
Calories: 367; Protein: 15.2 g; Carbohydrates: 66.5 g; Fat: 7.6 g; Fiber: 15 g

OTHER BENEFICIAL NUTRIENTS:
Excellent source of: vitamin A, vitamin C, vitamin B_6, folacin, zinc, fiber
Good source of: iron

ginger garlic tofu

INGREDIENTS

2 (12.3-oz.) pkgs. extra-firm, reduced-fat tofu

Extra-virgin olive oil cooking spray

1 tsp. sesame oil

2 cups finely chopped onion

4 cloves garlic, pressed

3 Tbsp. peeled and grated fresh ginger

2 Tbsp. arrowroot

1½ cups water

¼ cup reduced-sodium soy sauce

2 Tbsp. wine vinegar

1 Tbsp. honey

⅔ cup chopped green onion (optional)

2 Tbsp. sesame seeds, toasted

DIRECTIONS

1 Preheat the oven to 350°F.

2 Cut the tofu into ½ x 3 x 2-inch slices and press with a heavy cutting board for 15 minutes to remove excess liquid.

3 Heat a large, heavy saucepan over medium heat and coat with cooking spray, then add the sesame oil and sauté the onions and garlic until translucent.

4 Add the ginger and cook for 5 minutes longer. Dissolve the arrowroot in the water, then add it to the onions along with the soy sauce, vinegar, and honey.

5 Bring the sauce to a boil over high heat, stirring constantly. Reduce the heat and simmer for 5–7 minutes, or until the sauce has thickened.

6 Pour a thin layer of sauce in the bottom of an 8x12-inch baking pan. Arrange half of the tofu slices in the dish, followed by a thin layer of sauce, a second layer of tofu, and a final layer of sauce.

7 Bake for 20–25 minutes, or until heated through and bubbling.

8 Garnish with chopped green onions (optional) and toasted sesame seeds. Serve immediately.

NUTRIENT INFORMATION
(serving size: 4 oz.):
Calories: 128; Protein: 8.5 g;
Carbohydrates: 14.2 g; Fat: 3.7 g;
Fiber: 2.2 g

OTHER BENEFICIAL NUTRIENTS:
Good source of: iron

STORAGE INSTRUCTIONS

Refrigerate promptly; may be frozen.

greek egg scramble

SERVINGS: 2

INGREDIENTS

Extra-virgin olive oil cooking spray

1 cup peeled and finely diced eggplant

1 tsp. NutriFit Mediterranean Salt Free Spice Blend

2 plum tomatoes, chopped

2 cups fat-free egg substitute

¼ cup feta cheese, crumbled

DIRECTIONS

Note: For each teaspoon of the NutriFit Mediterranean Salt Free Spice Blend you may substitute: ¼ tsp. basil, ¼ tsp. oregano, ¼ tsp. garlic powder, and ¼ tsp. black pepper.

1 Heat a small skillet. Coat with olive oil spray, add the eggplant and spice blend, and sauté until soft.

2 Add the tomatoes and cook for 1 minute more.

3 Add the egg substitute and stir into the vegetable mixture until the eggs are set.

4 Add the feta cheese and stir once to spread, but do not melt the cheese.

STORAGE INSTRUCTIONS

Refrigerate promptly; do not freeze.

NUTRIENT INFORMATION (serving size: 1⅓ cup):
Calories: 184; Protein: 28.1 g; Carbohydrates: 12.1 g; Fat: 2 g; Fiber: 2.5 g

OTHER BENEFICIAL NUTRIENTS:
Excellent source of: vitamin A, vitamin C
Good source of: folacin, fiber

greek feta salad

SERVINGS: 6

INGREDIENTS

3 large cucumbers, peeled, seeded, and diced

3 oz. reduced-fat feta cheese

3 Tbsp. lemon juice

1½ tsp. olive oil

1½ cups chopped tomatoes (3 medium)

1 cup canned reduced-sodium garbanzo beans, drained

¼ cup reduced-sodium V8 juice

4 Tbsp. reduced-sodium vegetable broth

1 Tbsp. dried mint

Fresh mint (optional)

4 cups spinach leaves, rinsed and trimmed

DIRECTIONS

1 Place the cucumbers in a colander and sprinkle with a pinch of salt, and let stand for 20 minutes to drain the excess liquid.

2 In a bowl, mash the cheese with a fork and mix with the lemon juice and oil.

3 Rinse the cucumbers and pat dry with paper towels. Combine the cucumbers, cheese mixture, tomatoes, beans, V8 juice, vegetable broth, and mint. Place the salad in a shallow dish and decorate it with whole fresh mint leaves (optional).

4 Serve the salad on a bed of spinach leaves. Refrigerated, the salad will keep for up to two days.

STORAGE INSTRUCTIONS

Refrigerate promptly; do not freeze.

NUTRIENT INFORMATION (serving size: 1 cup):
Calories: 124; Protein: 8.2 g; Carbohydrates: 19.5 g; Fat: 3.8 g; Fiber: 6.2 g

OTHER BENEFICIAL NUTRIENTS:
Excellent source of: vitamin A, vitamin C, folacin, fiber
Good source of: vitamin B$_6$, calcium, iron

greek pita pizza

SERVINGS: 1

INGREDIENTS

1 whole-wheat pita, cut into
4 wedges

1 tsp. extra-virgin olive oil

¼ tsp. NutriFit Mediterranean
Salt Free Spice Blend

1 oz. vegetarian sausage, cut
into ¼-inch rounds

1 tomato, peeled and chopped

1 tsp. julienned basil

2 oz. feta cheese

DIRECTIONS

Note: For each teaspoon of the NutriFit Mediterranean Salt Free Spice Blend you may substitute: ¼ tsp. basil, ¼ tsp. oregano, ¼ tsp. garlic powder, and ¼ tsp. black pepper.

1 Preheat the oven to broil. Place a rack in the upper third of the oven.

2 On a baking sheet, arrange the pita bread wedges. Using a pastry brush, brush the tops with half of the olive oil. Sprinkle with the spice blend and broil 6 inches away from the heat source for 1–2 minutes, until lightly browned. Turn the pita over and repeat. Remove from the oven.

3 Reduce the heat to 450°F. Top the pitas with the sausage, tomatoes, and basil.

4 Crumble the feta cheese over the top. Bake for 5–7 minutes, until lightly browned. Serve at once.

STORAGE INSTRUCTIONS

Do not freeze.

NUTRIENT INFORMATION (serving size: 4 wedges):
Calories: 360; Protein: 25.4 g; Carbohydrates: 36.4 g; Fat: 15.1 g;
Fiber: 8.1 g

OTHER BENEFICIAL NUTRIENTS:
Excellent source of: vitamin A, vitamin C, calcium, fiber
Good source of: folacin, iron

grilled chicken breast

SERVINGS: 3

INGREDIENTS

1 lb. boneless, skinless chicken breasts

¼ tsp. NutriFit Calypso Salt Free Spice Blend

DIRECTIONS

Note: For each teaspoon of the NutriFit Calypso Salt Free Spice Blend you may substitute: ½ tsp. ground chiles, ¼ tsp. cumin, ⅛ tsp. black pepper, and ⅛ tsp. garlic powder.

1 Season the chicken with the spice blend.

2 Grill for about 10 minutes, until the chicken is thoroughly cooked.

STORAGE INSTRUCTIONS

Refrigerate promptly; may be frozen.

NUTRIENT INFORMATION (serving size: 1 breast):
Calories: 169; Protein: 34.9 g; Carbohydrates: 0.4 g; Fat: 1.9 g; Fiber: 0 g

OTHER BENEFICIAL NUTRIENTS:
Excellent source of: vitamin B_6
Good source of: vitamin A, zinc

grilled chicken breast sandwich

SERVINGS: 3

INGREDIENTS

1 lb. boneless, skinless chicken breasts

¼ tsp. NutriFit Calypso Salt Free Spice Blend

Canola oil cooking spray

3 whole sprouted-wheat buns

3 whole lettuce leaves

1 tomato, cut into ½-inch slices

DIRECTIONS

Note: For each teaspoon of the NutriFit Calypso Salt Free Spice Blend you may substitute: ½ tsp. ground chiles, ¼ tsp. ground cumin, ⅛ tsp. black pepper, and ⅛ tsp. garlic powder.

1 Season the chicken with the spice blend.

2 Heat a nonstick grill pan or a grill and coat with cooking spray. Add the chicken and cook for 6–8 minutes on one side, then 2–5 minutes on the second side, until cooked through.

3 Serve each chicken breast in a sprouted-wheat bun with a lettuce leaf and two slices of tomato.

STORAGE INSTRUCTIONS

Refrigerate promptly; do not freeze.

NUTRIENT INFORMATION (serving size: 1 sandwich):
Calories: 328; Protein: 52.5 g; Carbohydrates: 8.3 g; Fat: 8 g; Fiber: 3 g

OTHER BENEFICIAL NUTRIENTS:
Excellent source of: vitamin A, vitamin C, vitamin B$_6$, folacin, calcium
Good source of: iron, zinc, fiber

grilled chicken caesar salad

SERVINGS: 3

INGREDIENTS

1 lb. boneless, skinless chicken breasts

1 tsp. NutriFit Mediterranean Salt Free Spice Blend

1 slice whole-wheat bread

Extra-virgin olive oil cooking spray

6 cups shredded romaine lettuce

¼ cup grated Parmesan cheese

¼ cup fat-free Caesar dressing

DIRECTIONS

Note: For each teaspoon of the NutriFit Mediterranean Salt Free Spice Blend you may substitute: ¼ tsp. basil, ¼ tsp. oregano, ¼ tsp. garlic powder, and ¼ tsp. black pepper.

1 Preheat the grill or broiler. Wash the chicken and dry it with paper towels. Season the chicken on both sides with the spice blend. Broil or grill the chicken for 7–10 minutes on one side, then 5 minutes on the second side, until cooked through.

2 Meanwhile, cut the bread into ½-inch cubes. Spray the cubes with cooking spray and toast the cubes in a non-stick skillet until crispy; set aside.

3 Arrange the lettuce on a serving platter.

4 When the chicken is cool, slice it across the grain into ½-inch thick slices. Arrange it over the lettuce, sprinkle with the cheese, and top with the bread cubes. Serve the salad with the dressing on the side.

STORAGE INSTRUCTIONS

Refrigerate promptly; do not freeze.

NUTRIENT INFORMATION (serving size: 1½ cups):
Calories: 328; Protein: 52.5 g; Carbohydrates: 8.3 g; Fat: 8 g; Fiber: 3 g

OTHER BENEFICIAL NUTRIENTS:
Excellent source of: vitamin A, vitamin C, vitamin B_6, folacin, calcium
Good source of: iron, zinc, fiber

grilled ham and cheese sandwich

SERVINGS: 1

INGREDIENTS

2 slices whole-wheat bread

1 tsp. trans fat–free light margarine or spread

¼ tsp. Dijon mustard

2 slices low-sodium ham

1 slice low-fat, low-sodium Swiss cheese

DIRECTIONS

1 Spread one side of each piece of the bread with the margarine. Spread the mustard over the other side of one of the pieces.

2 Heat a nonstick skillet, place the slice of bread with the mustard "buttered" side down in the skillet. Place the ham and cheese on the bread, then top with the other slice, "buttered" side up.

3 Cook until toasted on the first side, then turn carefully, and cook on the other side until lightly browned and the cheese is melted. Serve immediately.

STORAGE INSTRUCTIONS

Refrigerate promptly; do not freeze.

NUTRIENT INFORMATION (serving size: 1 sandwich):
Calories: 285; Protein: 26.2 g; Carbohydrates: 26.1 g; Fat: 8.6 g; Fiber: 6.4 g

OTHER BENEFICIAL NUTRIENTS:
Excellent source of: vitamin A, calcium, fiber
Good source of: folacin, iron, zinc

grilled salmon with jicama orange salsa

SERVINGS: 3

INGREDIENTS

1 large navel orange, peeled, seeded, and diced

⅔ cup finely diced jicama

1 lb. salmon fillet, cut into 8 small pieces

1 Tbsp. lemon juice

1 tsp. NutriFit Calypso Salt Free Spice Blend

1 tsp. extra-virgin olive oil

DIRECTIONS

Note: For each teaspoon of the NutriFit Calypso Salt Free Spice Blend you may substitute: ½ tsp. ground chiles, ¼ tsp. cumin, ⅛ tsp. black pepper, and ⅛ tsp. garlic powder.

1 In a small bowl, gently mix the orange and the jicama; set aside.

2 Wash the salmon and pat it dry with paper towels. Season the salmon with the lemon juice, spice blend, and olive oil. In a nonstick skillet that has been heated to medium-high temperature, sear the fish (panfry over high heat) for 1–2 minutes on each side. Turn fish carefully, as it is delicate and may fall apart.

3 Put one-third of the jicama salsa on each of three plates and place two pieces of the hot salmon alongside.

STORAGE INSTRUCTIONS

Refrigerate; do not freeze.

BODY AFTER BABY

NUTRIENT INFORMATION (serving size: 5 oz., or a piece about the size of a deck of cards):
Calories: 172; Protein: 22.8 g; Carbohydrates: 7.5 g; Fat: 5.4 g; Fiber: 2.2 g

OTHER BENEFICIAL NUTRIENTS:
Excellent source of: vitamin A, vitamin C, vitamin B_6
Good source of: folacin

grilled turkey breast sandwich

SERVINGS: 1

INGREDIENTS

2 slices whole-wheat bread

1 tsp. trans fat–free light
margarine or spread

3 oz. cooked turkey breast

2 thin slices tomato

½ oz. provolone cheese

DIRECTIONS

1 Spread one side of each piece of the bread with the margarine.

2 Heat a nonstick skillet, place one slice of bread "buttered" side down in the skillet. Place the turkey, tomato, cheese, and the second slice of bread "buttered" side up on top.

3 Cook until toasted on the first side, then turn carefully, and cook on the other side until lightly browned and the cheese is melted. Serve immediately.

STORAGE INSTRUCTIONS

Refrigerate promptly; do not freeze.

NUTRIENT INFORMATION (serving size: 1 sandwich):
Calories: 272; Protein: 30.6 g; Carbohydrates: 25.4 g; Fat: 5.5 g;
Fiber: 3.9 g

OTHER BENEFICIAL NUTRIENTS:
Excellent source of: vitamin A, vitamin B$_6$, folacin, zinc
Good source of: vitamin C, calcium, iron, fiber

grilled vegetable salad

SERVINGS: 2

INGREDIENTS

1 zucchini

1 small eggplant

½ red or green bell pepper

½ large red onion

2 Tbsp. fat-free Italian dressing

DIRECTIONS

1 Slice the vegetables 1¼ inch thick and place in a bowl. Pour the dressing over vegetables and mix. Marinate for about 30 minutes.

2 Grill the vegetables in a grill pan over medium-high heat until soft.

STORAGE INSTRUCTIONS

Refrigerate promptly; may be frozen.

NUTRIENT INFORMATION (serving size: ½ cup):
Calories: 48; Protein: 2.5 g; Carbohydrates: 10.5 g; Fat: 0.3 g; Fiber: 4 g

OTHER BENEFICIAL NUTRIENTS:
Excellent source of: vitamin A, vitamin C, folacin
Good source of: vitamin B_6, fiber

herb dip

SERVINGS: 8

INGREDIENTS

3 Tbsp. reduced-fat buttermilk

4 oz. fat-free cream cheese

1 tsp. snipped fresh chives

1 tsp. dill weed

DIRECTIONS

1 In a food processor or blender, combine all of the ingredients. Process until smooth.

2 Refrigerate for at least 1 hour before serving (if time permits).

STORAGE INSTRUCTIONS

Refrigerate promptly; do not freeze. Keeps up to ten days under refrigeration, if the buttermilk and cheese were fresh at the time the dip was prepared.

NUTRIENT INFORMATION (serving size: 2 Tbsp.):
Calories: 28; Protein: 4.3 g; Carbohydrates: 1.7 g; Fat: 0 g; Fiber: 0.4 g

OTHER BENEFICIAL NUTRIENTS:
Excellent source of: vitamin A
Good source of: calcium

hickory-baked pork chops

INGREDIENTS

1¼ lbs. center-cut loin pork chops, trimmed of fat (4)

1 (18-oz.) can stewed tomatoes

1 small onion, thinly sliced

1 clove garlic, minced

1 tsp. oregano

1 (8-oz.) can reduced-sodium tomato sauce

2 Tbsp. hickory smoke–flavored barbecue sauce

Chopped parsley (optional)

DIRECTIONS

1 Preheat the oven to 350°F.

2 Rinse the pork chops and pat them dry with paper towels.

3 In a shallow 2-quart casserole, stir together the tomatoes, onion, garlic, oregano, tomato sauce, and barbecue sauce. Add the pork chops and spoon half of the tomato mixture over them.

4 Cover the casserole and bake until the chops are done (20–30 minutes, depending on the thickness of the chops).

5 Sprinkle with the chopped parsley before serving (optional).

STORAGE INSTRUCTIONS

Refrigerate promptly; may be frozen.

NUTRIENT INFORMATION (serving size: 1 chop):
Calories: 230; Protein: 26.2 g; Carbohydrates: 13.7 g; Fat: 7.2 g; Fiber: 1.6 g

OTHER BENEFICIAL NUTRIENTS:
Excellent source of: vitamin A, vitamin C, vitamin B_6, zinc
Good source of: iron

high-protein french toast

INGREDIENTS

2 cups fat-free cottage cheese

⅛ tsp. cinnamon

3 cups fat-free egg substitute

6 slices whole-wheat cinnamon bread

Canola oil cooking spray

Syrup or honey (optional)

DIRECTIONS

1 In a food processor, process the cottage cheese and cinnamon until smooth. Add the egg substitute and stir well.

2 Arrange the bread slices in a shallow dish. Pour the egg mixture over the bread and soak the slices with the mixture.

3 Heat a flat griddle, coat with cooking spray, and cook the slices until golden brown on one side, then turn and cook them on the other side until done. Serve with syrup or honey (optional).

STORAGE INSTRUCTIONS

Refrigerate promptly; may be frozen.

NUTRIENT INFORMATION (serving size: 1 slice):
Calories: 134; Protein: 14.4 g; Carbohydrates: 15.7 g; Fat: 0.9 g; Fiber: 0.6 g

OTHER BENEFICIAL NUTRIENTS:
Excellent source of: vitamin A
Good source of: vitamin B_6

holiday cheese log

INGREDIENTS

4 oz. fat-free cream cheese

2 cups shredded reduced-fat cheddar cheese

3 oz. reduced-fat spiced cream cheese

1 tsp. Worcestershire sauce

1 tsp. NutriFit Calypso Salt Free Spice Blend

2 drops Tabasco sauce

2 tsp. sesame seeds, toasted

Cilantro leaves and parsley sprigs (garnish)

DIRECTIONS

Note: For each teaspoon of the NutriFit Calypso Salt Free Spice Blend you may substitute: ½ tsp. ground chiles, ¼ tsp. cumin, ⅛ tsp. black pepper, and ⅛ tsp. garlic powder.

1 In a food processor, combine the cream cheese, cheddar cheese, and spiced cream cheese and process until smooth.

2 Add the Worcestershire sauce, spice blend, and Tabasco and process with short bursts to blend. Taste for seasoning. Remove the mixture to a piece of waxed paper.

3 Form the mixture into a log and roll it in the toasted sesame seeds, using the waxed paper to help roll the log or ball. Refrigerate until ready to serve, then garnish with cilantro and parsley. If desired, you can roll the log in Grape-Nuts instead of the seeds, or a combination of both seeds and cereal.

STORAGE INSTRUCTIONS

Refrigerate promptly; do not freeze.

NUTRIENT INFORMATION (serving size: 1½ oz., or one 2-inch piece):
Calories: 25; Protein: 3.7 g; Carbohydrates: 0.5 g; Fat: 0.9 g; Fiber: 0 g

OTHER BENEFICIAL NUTRIENTS:
Good source of: vitamin A

honey balsamic vinaigrette dressing

3 CUPS

INGREDIENTS

¼ cup honey

½ cup canned apricots, drained

⅓ cup balsamic or red-wine vinegar

2 tsp. Dijon mustard

1 clove garlic, minced

1 tsp. NutriFit Mediterranean Salt Free Spice Blend

¼ tsp. salt

1 Tbsp. olive oil

DIRECTIONS

Note: For each teaspoon of the NutriFit Mediterranean Salt Free Spice Blend, you may substitute: ¼ tsp. basil, ¼ tsp. oregano, ¼ tsp. garlic powder, and ¼ tsp. black pepper.

1 In a small glass bowl, heat the honey in a microwave oven until it liquefies.

2 In a food processor, combine the honey, apricots, vinegar, mustard, garlic, spice blend, and salt and blend until smooth. With the motor running, slowly drizzle in olive oil until the dressing thickens and is well combined.

STORAGE INSTRUCTIONS

Refrigerate promptly; do not freeze. Refrigerated, this dressing will remain fresh for about two weeks.

NUTRIENT INFORMATION (serving size: 1 Tbsp.):
Calories: 10; Protein: 0 g; Carbohydrates: 3 g; Fat: 0 g; Fiber: 0 g

huevos rancheros

SERVINGS: 1

INGREDIENTS

1 tsp. olive oil

1 tsp. finely chopped onion

2 Tbsp. chopped tomato

1 tsp. fresh salsa, medium-spicy

½ tsp. chopped cilantro

2 eggs

Salt (optional)

DIRECTIONS

1 Heat a nonstick skillet over medium heat. Add the oil and onion and sauté until the onion is soft. Add the tomato, salsa, and cilantro and cook 1 minute more. Remove the mixture from the skillet; set aside.

2 Add the eggs and cook, yolk side up, for 2 minutes. Season with a pinch of salt (optional).

3 Add the reserved sauce and finish cooking, uncovered. Serve immediately.

STORAGE INSTRUCTIONS

Refrigerate promptly; do not freeze.

NUTRIENT INFORMATION (serving size: 2 eggs):
Calories: 196; Protein: 13.1 g; Carbohydrates: 2.9 g; Fat: 14.6 g; Fiber: 0.5 g

OTHER BENEFICIAL NUTRIENTS:
Excellent source of: vitamin A, folacin
Good source of: vitamin C, iron

ipanema wrap

SERVINGS: 4

INGREDIENTS

2 Granny Smith apples

¾ cup diced ham

1 cup diced, cooked chicken breast

1 cup baby corn, drained and cut into ½-inch pieces

½ cup green olives, pitted, slivered, and well rinsed

¼ cup raisins

4 celery stalks, thinly sliced

2 Tbsp. fat-free mayonnaise

1 tsp. mustard

1 tsp. NutriFit Calypso Salt Free Spice Blend

1 piece lavosh or whole-wheat tortilla

DIRECTIONS

Note: For each teaspoon of the NutriFit Calypso Salt Free Spice Blend you may substitute: ½ tsp. ground chiles, ¼ tsp. cumin, ⅛ tsp. black pepper, and ⅛ tsp. garlic powder.

1 Wash the apples, but do not peel. Cut into ½-inch dice.

2 In a large bowl, gently mix the apples, ham, chicken, corn, olives, raisins, and celery.

3 In a small bowl, combine the mayonnaise, mustard, and spice blend. Add to the apple mixture and chill before serving.

4 Wrap in lavosh or whole-wheat tortilla (or serve on a bed of greens).

STORAGE INSTRUCTIONS

Best eaten within two days; do not freeze.

NUTRIENT INFORMATION (serving size: 1 wrap):
Calories: 410; Protein: 14.8 g; Carbohydrates: 44.7 g; Fat: 20.1 g; Fiber: 6.7 g

OTHER BENEFICIAL NUTRIENTS:
Excellent source of: vitamin A, vitamin C, vitamin B$_6$, folacin, calcium, fiber
Good source of: iron

kale and millet stew

SERVINGS: 4

INGREDIENTS

1 Tbsp. canola oil

½ cup chopped onion

1 small butternut squash, peeled, seeded, and cut into 1-inch cubes (1 cup)

1 cup millet, rinsed and drained

3 cups water

1 Tbsp. NutriFit Lemon Garden Salt Free Spice Blend

1 Tbsp. reduced-sodium soy sauce

1 bunch kale, shredded

DIRECTIONS

Note: For each tablespoon of the NutriFit Lemon Garden Salt Free Spice Blend you may substitute: ½ tsp. basil, ½ tsp. marjoram, ½ tsp. black pepper, and ½ tsp. dill weed.

1 Heat a medium saucepan. Add the oil, and sauté the onion.

2 Add the squash, millet, water, spice blend, and soy sauce. Bring to a boil, cover, and cook for 35–45 minutes. Stir to mix. Add the kale and let stand for 10 minutes before serving.

STORAGE INSTRUCTIONS

Refrigerate promptly; may be frozen.

NUTRIENT INFORMATION (serving size: 1½ cups):
Calories: 390; Protein: 11.6 g; Carbohydrates: 68.5 g; Fat: 8.3 g; Fiber: 11.9 g

OTHER BENEFICIAL NUTRIENTS:
Excellent source of: vitamin A, vitamin C, vitamin B_6, folacin, calcium, fiber
Good source of: iron, zinc

lasagna roll-ups

SERVINGS: 2

INGREDIENTS

4 large red Swiss chard leaves, steamed

1 cup reduced-fat ricotta cheese

½ tsp. NutriFit Mediterranean Salt Free Spice Blend

¼ cup grated Parmesan cheese

6 whole lasagna noodles, cooked according to package directions

1 cup marinara sauce

DIRECTIONS

Note: For each teaspoon of the NutriFit Mediterranean Salt Free Spice Blend you may substitute: ¼ tsp. basil, ¼ tsp. oregano, ¼ tsp. black pepper, and ¼ tsp. garlic powder.

1 Preheat the oven to 375°F.

2 In a food processor, combine the chard, ricotta cheese, spice blend, and half of the Parmesan cheese. Process using short on/off bursts, just until blended.

3 Lay out the lasagna noodles. Spread the mixture evenly over the length of each noodle, leaving 1 inch free at one end of each noodle. Roll the lasagna noodles. Place in a large baking dish. Spoon marinara sauce over the top, and sprinkle with the remaining Parmesan cheese. Bake for 20 minutes, or until heated through.

STORAGE INSTRUCTIONS

Refrigerate promptly; may be frozen.

NUTRIENT INFORMATION (serving size: 1½ roll-ups):
Calories: 426; Protein: 23.2 g; Carbohydrates: 56.7 g; Fat: 9.7 g; Fiber: 2.9 g

OTHER BENEFICIAL NUTRIENTS:
Excellent source of: vitamin A, vitamin C, calcium
Good source of: iron, fiber

lavosh wrap with hummus and veggies

SERVINGS: 1

INGREDIENTS

1 Tbsp. hummus

¼ piece lavosh

½ cup alfalfa sprouts

½ cucumber, thinly sliced

¼ cup baby carrots

DIRECTIONS

1 Spread the hummus lengthwise on the lavosh.

2 Place a row of sprouts horizontally over the hummus, then do the same with the cucumbers.

3 Wrap up the lavosh.

4 Serve with carrots on the side.

STORAGE INSTRUCTIONS

Refrigerate promptly; do not freeze.

BODY AFTER BABY

NUTRIENT INFORMATION (serving size: 1 wrap):
Calories: 110; Protein: 6.4 g; Carbohydrates: 18.2 g; Fat: 1.3 g; Fiber: 3.5 g

OTHER BENEFICIAL NUTRIENTS:
Excellent source of: vitamin A, vitamin C, folacin
Good source of: fiber

lemon basil chicken

SERVINGS: 4

INGREDIENTS

4 (4-oz.) boneless, skinless chicken breasts

1 tsp. NutriFit Mediterranean Salt Free Spice Blend

2 tsp. olive oil

½ cup reduced-sodium chicken broth

2 Tbsp. lemon juice

2 tsp. grated lemon peel

3 Tbsp. chopped basil

Basil leaves (optional)

DIRECTIONS

Note: For each teaspoon of the NutriFit Mediterranean Salt Free Spice Blend you may substitute: ¼ tsp. basil, ¼ tsp. oregano, ¼ tsp. garlic powder, and ¼ tsp. black pepper.

1 Wash the chicken and pat it dry. Season on both sides with the spice blend.

2 Heat a large nonstick skillet and add 1 tsp. of the oil. Cook the chicken for about 3 minutes on each side, until lightly browned on both sides. Add the broth, lemon juice, and lemon peel. Reduce the heat, cover, and simmer until the chicken is no longer pink in the center. Remove the chicken to a warm platter.

3 Bring the cooking liquid to a boil over high heat; boil until the liquid is reduced by about two-thirds. Add the basil, any accumulated juices from the chicken, then the remaining oil. Reduce the heat slightly and boil gently until it thickens. Pour the sauce around the chicken, and garnish with additional basil leaves (optional).

STORAGE INSTRUCTIONS

Refrigerate promptly; may be frozen.

NUTRIENT INFORMATION (serving size: 1 breast):
Calories: 204; Protein: 39.6 g; Carbohydrates: 4.3 g; Fat: 2.2 g; Fiber: 0.6 g

OTHER BENEFICIAL NUTRIENTS:
Excellent source of: vitamin A, vitamin C, vitamin B_6
Good source of: zinc

lemon-grilled london broil

SERVINGS: 6

INGREDIENTS

2 lbs. top round steak

¼ cup pureed papaya

Meat tenderizer (optional)

¼ cup extra-virgin olive oil

2 tsp. lemon juice

1 tsp. NutriFit Mediterranean Salt Free Spice Blend

1 tsp. lemon pepper

2 cloves garlic, minced

4 tsp. chopped parsley

2 tsp. tarragon vinegar

DIRECTIONS

Note: For each teaspoon of the NutriFit Mediterranean Salt Free Spice Blend you may substitute: ¼ tsp. basil, ¼ tsp. oregano, ¼ tsp. garlic powder, and ¼ tsp. black pepper.

1 Score the top and bottom of the steak with a 1½-inch square pattern, and score the side. Sprinkle the meat liberally with pureed papaya, then pierce with a fork ⅛ inch apart and at least halfway through the meat on both sides. Sprinkle lightly with water and rub in tenderizer (optional). Place on a plate; cover and let stand for 1 hour.

2 In a small bowl, mix together the oil, lemon juice, spice blend, lemon pepper, garlic, parsley, and vinegar. Pour the marinade over the meat, reserving a portion to be used for brushing. Cover the dish and refrigerate for 3 hours, turning every half hour.

3 Preheat the grill for hot heat.

4 Lightly oil the grate, and place the meat on the grill. Cook for 5 minutes. Turn the meat over, brush with marinade, and cook for another 5 minutes. Cut in thin strips across the grain.

STORAGE INSTRUCTIONS

Best eaten within two days; may be frozen.

NUTRIENT INFORMATION (serving size: 5 oz., a piece about the size of a deck of playing cards):
Calories: 260; Protein: 35 g; Carbohydrates: 0.7 g; Fat: 12.2 g; Fiber: 0.1 g

OTHER BENEFICIAL NUTRIENTS:
Excellent source of: vitamin B_6, zinc
Good source of: vitamin A, iron

lemon rice

SERVINGS: 6

INGREDIENTS

1 tsp. extra-virgin olive oil

1 clove garlic, minced

1 cup uncooked brown rice

1 tsp. grated lemon peel

¼ tsp. white pepper

2 cups reduced-sodium chicken broth

2 Tbsp. chopped parsley

DIRECTIONS

1 Heat a medium-size saucepan over medium heat. Add the oil and sauté the garlic for 1 minute, or until soft.

2 Add the rice, lemon peel, pepper, and broth and bring the mixture to a boil, stirring once or twice. Lower the heat to a simmer and cover with a tight-fitting lid. Cook for 15 minutes, or until the liquid is absorbed. Stir in the parsley and serve hot.

STORAGE INSTRUCTIONS:

Refrigerate promptly; may be frozen.

NUTRIENT INFORMATION (serving size: ½ cup):
Calories: 127; Protein: 3.8 g; Carbohydrates: 26 g; Fat: 0.7 g; Fiber: 0.5 g

OTHER BENEFICIAL NUTRIENTS:
Excellent source of: vitamin A
Good source of: vitamin C, iron

lentil pilaf

INGREDIENTS

1 Tbsp. extra-virgin olive oil

½ cup uncooked vermicelli, finely broken up

2 cloves garlic, minced

2 Tbsp. diced onion

1 cup uncooked long-grain brown rice

1¼ cups reduced-sodium vegetable broth

1¼ cups hot water

1 tsp. NutriFit Calypso Salt Free Spice Blend

1 whole bay leaf

1 cup lentils, cooked

2 Tbsp. grated fat-free Parmesan cheese

¼ cup chopped Italian parsley

DIRECTIONS

Note: For each teaspoon of the NutriFit Calypso Salt Free Spice Blend you may substitute: ½ tsp. ground chiles, ¼ tsp. cumin, ⅛ tsp. black pepper, and ⅛ tsp. garlic powder.

1 Heat the oil in a large skillet, and sauté the vermicelli, garlic, and onion until golden brown.

2 Add the rice, broth, hot water, spice blend, and bay leaf. Cover and simmer for 15–20 minutes.

3 Add the lentils to the rice and stir until warmed through. Fluff the rice with a fork and remove the bay leaf. Sprinkle with the cheese and the parsley and serve immediately.

STORAGE INSTRUCTIONS

Refrigerate promptly; may be frozen.

NUTRIENT INFORMATION (serving size: 1 cup):
Calories: 210; Protein: 7.4 g; Carbohydrates: 38.4 g; Fat: 2.7 g; Fiber: 3.6 g

OTHER BENEFICIAL NUTRIENTS:
Excellent source of: vitamin A, folacin
Good source of: vitamin B_6, iron, fiber

linguine with shrimp

SERVINGS: 4

INGREDIENTS

1½ oz. sun-dried tomatoes, packed without oil

8 oz. uncooked linguine

Extra-virgin olive oil cooking spray

1 lb. medium shrimp, peeled and deveined

½ cup finely chopped green onions

1 clove garlic, minced

½ cup dry white wine

3 Tbsp. lemon juice

1 Tbsp. capers, drained

1 Tbsp. olive oil

1 tsp. NutriFit Mediterranean Salt Free Spice Blend

Black pepper (optional)

½ cup grated fat-free Parmesan cheese

DIRECTIONS

Note: For each teaspoon of the NutriFit Mediterranean Salt Free Spice Blend you may substitute: ¼ tsp. basil, ¼ tsp. oregano, ¼ tsp. garlic powder, and ¼ tsp. black pepper.

1 In a bowl, combine the sun-dried tomatoes with ½ cup boiling water. Let stand for 30 minutes, then drain well. Slice thinly and set aside. Cook the pasta according to package directions, omitting the salt and fat; set aside.

2 Heat a large nonstick skillet over medium-high heat until hot. Coat with extra-virgin olive oil cooking spray and add the shrimp and green onions; sauté for 5 minutes, or until the shrimp are done. Add the sun-dried tomatoes, garlic, wine, lemon juice, capers, olive oil, and spice blend. Cook for 1 minute, or until thoroughly heated. Add a dash of black pepper (optional).

3 Remove the shrimp mixture from the heat, and add the cooked pasta; toss well. Serve with cheese.

STORAGE INSTRUCTIONS

Refrigerate promptly; do not freeze.

NUTRIENT INFORMATION (serving size: 1¼ cups):
Calories: 338; Protein: 26 g; Carbohydrates: 41.1 g; Fat: 4.8 g; Fiber: 1.9 g

OTHER BENEFICIAL NUTRIENTS:
Excellent source of: vitamin A, vitamin C
Good source of: vitamin B$_6$, calcium, iron, zinc

maple walnut pudding

INGREDIENTS

12 oz. extra-firm reduced-fat tofu

½ cup reduced-fat vanilla soy milk

3 Tbsp. trans fat–free light margarine or spread, melted

⅓ cup maple syrup

⅓ cup walnuts, ground

1 tsp. lemon juice

3 Tbsp. grated lemon peel

1 tsp. vanilla extract

DIRECTIONS

1 In a blender or food processor, combine all the ingredients and process until smooth.

2 Chill for 2 to 4 hours.

STORAGE INSTRUCTIONS

Refrigerate promptly; do not freeze.

NUTRIENT INFORMATION (serving size: ½ cup):
Calories: 177; Protein: 6.1 g; Carbohydrates: 16.3 g; Fat: 10.4 g; Fiber: 1.3 g

OTHER BENEFICIAL NUTRIENTS:
Excellent source of: vitamin A

mexican hot cocoa

INGREDIENTS

¼ cup sugar

¼ cup unsweetened cocoa powder

¼ cup water

¼ tsp. NutriFit Certainly Cinnamon Salt Free Spice Blend

2 cups fat-free milk

¼ tsp. vanilla extract

⅛ tsp. almond extract

DIRECTIONS

Note: For each teaspoon of the NutriFit Certainly Cinnamon Salt Free Blend you may substitute: ½ tsp. cinnamon, ¼ tsp. nutmeg, ⅛ tsp. ginger, and ⅛ tsp. cloves.

1 In a small saucepan, combine the sugar, cocoa, water, and spice blend. Bring to a boil over medium-high heat, stirring until the sugar and cocoa are completely dissolved. Stir in the milk, then stir over medium heat until just steaming; do not boil.

2 Remove the pan from the heat and stir in the vanilla and almond extracts.

3 Pour half the hot milk mixture into a blender and whirl until very frothy; pour into mugs and serve at once. Repeat with the remaining mixture.

STORAGE INSTRUCTIONS

Best eaten within two days; do not freeze.

NUTRIENT INFORMATION (serving size: ⅔ cup):
Calories: 119; Protein: 6.9 g; Carbohydrates: 24.2 g; Fat: 1 g; Fiber: 1.4 g

OTHER BENEFICIAL NUTRIENTS:
Excellent source of: vitamin A, calcium

oatmeal chocolate chip cookies

YIELD: ABOUT 4 DOZEN

INGREDIENTS

Canola oil cooking spray

¼ cup fat-free egg substitute

1 cup packed brown sugar

2 Tbsp. canola oil

¾ cup plain fat-free yogurt

2 tsp. vanilla extract

2 cups old-fashioned rolled oats

1½ cups unbleached
all-purpose flour

1 tsp. baking soda

1 tsp. NutriFit Certainly
Cinnamon Salt Free Spice Blend

¼ tsp. salt

½ cup mini chocolate chips

DIRECTIONS

Note: For each teaspoon of the NutriFit Certainly Cinnamon Salt Free Spice Blend you may substitute: ½ tsp. cinnamon, ¼ tsp. nutmeg, ⅛ tsp. ginger, and ⅛ tsp. cloves.

1 Preheat the oven to 350°F. Coat two baking sheets with cooking spray.

2 In a large bowl, beat the egg substitute, brown sugar, and oil with an electric mixer until smooth and thickened. Add the yogurt and vanilla and beat again. Add the oats, flour, baking soda, spice blend, and salt; beat until well mixed. Stir in the chocolate chips.

3 Drop the batter by rounded teaspoonfuls onto the baking sheets about 2 inches apart. Bake for 10–12 minutes, or until the cookies are lightly browned. Cool on a wire rack.

STORAGE INSTRUCTIONS

Store at room temperature; may be frozen.

NUTRIENT INFORMATION (serving size: 1 cookie):
Calories: 74; Protein: 1.5 g; Carbohydrates: 15 g; Fat: 1.1 g; Fiber: 0.7 g

open-faced turkey club sandwich

SERVINGS: 1

INGREDIENTS

1 slice turkey bacon

3 oz. cooked turkey breast

½ tomato, thinly sliced

1 romaine lettuce leaf

1 slice whole-wheat bread

DIRECTIONS

1 Cook the turkey bacon until crisp. Drain and cut the slice in half; set aside.

2 Slice the turkey breast thin. Assemble the sandwich by wrapping the turkey breast, bacon, and tomato slices in the lettuce leaf, which has been washed and patted dry.

3 If serving at a later time, put the bread in a bag on the side. Assemble the sandwich open-faced, putting the turkey breast on the bread, topping with crisscrossed bacon and tomato slices.

You may put condiments (mayonnaise and/or mustard) on the side.

STORAGE INSTRUCTIONS

Refrigerate promptly; do not freeze.

NUTRIENT INFORMATION (serving size: 1 sandwich):
Calories: 224; Protein: 31 g; Carbohydrates: 15 g; Fat: 4.4 g; Fiber: 2.9 g

OTHER BENEFICIAL NUTRIENTS:
Excellent source of: vitamin A, vitamin C, vitamin B$_6$, folacin
Good source of: iron, zinc, fiber

oriental beef with peppers

INGREDIENTS

1 cup shiitake mushrooms

1 tsp. cornstarch

¼ cup reduced-sodium beef broth

1 Tbsp. reduced-sodium soy sauce

1 tsp. sesame oil

1 lb. sirloin steak

1¼ Tbsp. canola oil

1 clove garlic, minced

¼ tsp. Chinese five-spice powder

2 small onions, cut into wedges

1 medium red bell pepper, thinly sliced

1 medium green bell pepper, thinly sliced

DIRECTIONS

1 If using dried shiitake mushrooms, place 1 oz. mushrooms in a medium bowl; add enough warm water to cover the mushrooms completely. Let stand for 30 minutes; drain. Squeeze excess water from the mushrooms. Remove and discard the stems. Slice the caps into thin strips.

2 If using fresh mushrooms, discard the stems from 1 cup mushrooms. Slice the caps into thin strips.

3 In a small bowl, combine the cornstarch, broth, soy sauce, and sesame oil; set aside.

4 Cut the meat into thin slices, each about 1 inch long.

5 Heat a wok or large skillet over high heat, add the canola oil, garlic, and five-spice powder; stir-fry for 15 seconds.

6 Add the meat to the wok; stir-fry about 5 minutes, until browned. Add the onions; stir fry for 2 minutes. Add the mushrooms and peppers; stir-fry for about 2 minutes, until the peppers are crisp-tender.

7 Stir the cornstarch mixture; add to the wok. Cook and stir until the liquid boils and thickens.

STORAGE INSTRUCTIONS

Refrigerate promptly; may be frozen.

NUTRIENT INFORMATION (serving size: 1¼ cups):
Calories: 415; Protein: 30.7 g; Carbohydrates: 40.8 g; Fat: 14 g; Fiber: 4.2 g

OTHER BENEFICIAL NUTRIENTS:
Excellent source of: vitamin A, vitamin C, vitamin B_6, folacin, zinc
Good source of: iron, fiber

oriental red snapper

INGREDIENTS

4 (6-oz.) red snapper fillets

½ cup thinly sliced green onion

1½ Tbsp. peeled and minced fresh ginger

1 tsp. sugar

½ tsp. dried crushed red pepper

2 cloves garlic, crushed

1 Tbsp. reduced-sodium soy sauce

2 Tbsp. unsweetened pineapple juice

1 tsp. sesame oil

DIRECTIONS

1 Wash the fish fillets and pat dry with paper towels. Place the fillets in a shallow dish; set aside.

2 In a small bowl, combine the green onions, ginger, sugar, red pepper, garlic, soy sauce, pineapple juice, and sesame oil. Spread the green onion mixture evenly over the fillets. Cover and marinate in the refrigerator for 30 minutes.

3 Line a steaming basket with a plate at least 1 inch smaller in diameter than the basket. Transfer the fillets to the plate, using a slotted spoon; discard the marinade. Place the steaming basket over boiling water. Cover and steam for 10 minutes, or until the fish flakes easily when tested with a fork.

STORAGE INSTRUCTIONS

Best eaten within two days; do not freeze.

NUTRIENT INFORMATION (serving size: 1 fillet):
Calories: 203; Protein: 35.6 g; Carbohydrates: 5.1 g; Fat: 3.5 g; Fiber: 0.5 g

OTHER BENEFICIAL NUTRIENTS:
Excellent source of: vitamin A, vitamin B_6

pasta with black beans

SERVINGS: 6

INGREDIENTS

1 (28-oz.) can reduced-sodium Italian tomatoes with liquid, chopped

3 cloves garlic, minced

1 cup chopped onion

¼ cup diced seeded green chiles (you may use canned)

1 large bell pepper, chopped

1 tsp. NutriFit Calypso Salt Free Spice Blend

2 cups cooked black beans

1 cup fresh tomato salsa

4 cups dry pasta, cooked al dente and drained

DIRECTIONS

Note: For each teaspoon of the NutriFit Calypso Salt Free Spice Blend you may substitute: ½ tsp. ground chiles, ¼ tsp. ground cumin, ⅛ tsp. black pepper, and ⅛ garlic powder.

1 In a large saucepan, heat the liquid from the tomatoes. Add the garlic, onions, green chiles, and bell pepper. Cook until the onions are translucent.

2 Add the spice blend, black beans, salsa, and tomatoes. When the sauce comes to a boil, reduce the heat and cook for 20 minutes.

3 Add the cooked pasta and cook for 5 minutes more.

STORAGE INSTRUCTIONS

Refrigerate promptly; may be frozen.

NUTRIENT INFORMATION (serving size: 1½ cups):
Calories: 285; Protein: 15.2 g; Carbohydrates: 54.2 g; Fat: 1.3 g; Fiber: 9.7 g

OTHER BENEFICIAL NUTRIENTS:
Excellent source of: vitamin A, vitamin C, folacin, fiber
Good source of: vitamin B$_6$, iron, zinc

pasta with dilled pea sauce

INGREDIENTS

1 tsp. extra-virgin olive oil

1 clove garlic, peeled and finely chopped

1 leek, thinly sliced

3 cups reduced-sodium vegetable broth

¼ cup fresh dill

3 cups frozen peas

2 Tbsp. cornstarch

4 Tbsp. water

8 oz. uncooked dry pasta

¼ tsp. salt

Dash hot pepper sauce (optional)

DIRECTIONS

1 Heat a medium saucepan over medium-high heat, add the oil and the garlic, and cook for 2 minutes.

2 Add the leek and cook for 3 minutes more.

3 Stir in the vegetable broth and dill, and bring to a boil. Add half the peas and bring back to a boil.

4 Remove the sauce from the heat. Pour the mixture into a blender and puree until smooth.

5 Mix the cornstarch and water until the cornstarch dissolves. Add it to the sauce, return it to the heat, and stir until bubbling and thickened. Stir in the remaining peas.

6 Cook the pasta according to the package directions, drain, and transfer to a large warm bowl.

7 To serve, add the salt and hot pepper sauce (optional) to the pea sauce; toss with the pasta.

STORAGE INSTRUCTIONS

Refrigerate promptly; may be frozen.

NUTRIENT INFORMATION (serving size: 1 cup):
Calories: 374; Protein: 14.6 g; Carbohydrates: 73.4 g; Fat: 2.5 g; Fiber: 8.6 g

OTHER BENEFICIAL NUTRIENTS:
Excellent source of: vitamin A, vitamin C, iron, fiber
Good source of: vitamin B_6, folacin, zinc

pasta with turkey meat sauce

SERVINGS: 4

INGREDIENTS

2 tsp. olive oil

½ cup chopped onion

1 clove garlic, finely chopped

1 lb. ground turkey

1 Tbsp. NutriFit Mediterranean Salt Free Spice Blend

1 (28-oz.) can crushed tomatoes

½ tsp. sugar (optional)

¼ cup red wine

8 oz. dry pasta, cooked according to package directions

DIRECTIONS

Note: For each tablespoon of the NutriFit Mediterranean Salt Free Spice Blend you may substitute: 1 tsp. basil, 1 tsp. oregano, ½ tsp. black pepper, and ½ tsp. garlic powder.

1 Heat a nonstick saucepan, add the olive oil, and add the onion and cook until translucent, but not brown, stirring constantly. Add the garlic and cook for 1 minute more.

2 Add the ground turkey and spice blend and brown well, stirring to break up chunks of meat. Drain off the excess liquid.

3 Add the tomatoes and stir well. Correct the seasoning (add more spice blend and the sugar, if needed). Reduce the heat to low, cover, and simmer 20–30 minutes, stirring occasionally.

4 Add the wine and cook for 10 minutes more, uncovered. Serve over the hot pasta.

STORAGE INSTRUCTIONS

Refrigerate promptly; may be frozen.

NUTRIENT INFORMATION (serving size: 1 cup pasta and ½ cup sauce):
Calories: 486; Protein: 34.3 g; Carbohydrates: 59.7 g; Fat: 11.3 g; Fiber: 5.1 g

OTHER BENEFICIAL NUTRIENTS:
Excellent source of: vitamin A, vitamin C, fiber
Good source of: calcium, iron

pasta with vegetarian meatballs

SERVINGS: 4

INGREDIENTS

12 oz. ground meat alternative

1 Tbsp. NutriFit Mediterranean Salt Free Spice Blend

½ cup chopped onions

2 cloves garlic, chopped

1 cup quick-cooking rolled oats

½ cup fat-free egg substitute

2 cups marinara sauce

8 oz. dry pasta, cooked according to package directions

DIRECTIONS

Note: For each tablespoon of the NutriFit Mediterranean Salt Free Spice Blend you may substitute: 1 tsp. basil, 1 tsp. oregano, ½ tsp. black pepper, and ½ tsp. garlic powder.

1 In a large bowl, combine the ground meat alternative, spice blend, onions, garlic, quick oats, and egg substitute. Roll the mixture into 2-inch balls (should yield approximately 20).

2 In a nonstick skillet, brown the meatballs over medium-high heat, shaking the pan frequently to prevent sticking.

3 Heat the marinara sauce and combine with the pasta and veggie meatballs.

STORAGE INSTRUCTIONS

Refrigerate promptly; may be frozen.

NUTRIENT INFORMATION (serving size: 1 cup pasta and 5 meatballs):
Calories: 440; Protein: 26.6 g; Carbohydrates: 74.5 g; Fat: 3.3 g; Fiber: 6.5 g

OTHER BENEFICIAL NUTRIENTS:
Excellent source of: vitamin A, fiber
Good source of: folacin, iron, zinc

pasta with white beans

INGREDIENTS

1 (28-oz.) can Italian plum tomatoes, drained, reserving liquid

1 cup chopped onion

3 cloves garlic, minced

1 large carrot, finely chopped

2 cups dried white beans, cooked and drained

2 Tbsp. dried currants

2 tsp. NutriFit Mediterranean Salt Free Spice Blend

2 cups dry pasta, cooked according to package directions

Fat-free Parmesan cheese (optional)

DIRECTIONS

Note: For each teaspoon of the NutriFit Mediterranean Salt Free Spice Blend you may substitute: ¼ tsp. basil, ¼ tsp. oregano, ¼ tsp. garlic powder, and ¼ tsp. black pepper.

1 In a large stockpot, heat the reserved tomato liquid. Add the onion, garlic, and carrots and cook for 2–3 minutes, until the onion begins to soften, stirring often. Stir in the beans, currants, spice blend, and tomatoes. Bring the mixture to a boil; reduce the heat, cover, and cook gently until the carrots are tender, about 10 minutes.

2 Stir in the cooked pasta and heat for about 5 minutes. Serve with fat-free Parmesan cheese on the side (optional).

STORAGE INSTRUCTIONS

Refrigerate promptly; may be frozen.

NUTRIENT INFORMATION (serving size: 2 cups):
Calories: 365; Protein: 15.8 g; Carbohydrates: 71 g; Fat: 1.3 g; Fiber: 12.6 g

OTHER BENEFICIAL NUTRIENTS:
Excellent source of: vitamin C, folacin, fiber
Good source of: vitamin B_6, calcium, iron, zinc

peach and berry crisp

INGREDIENTS

8 medium firm, ripe peaches

⅓ cup granulated sugar

2 Tbsp. lemon juice

½ tsp. NutriFit Certainly Cinnamon Salt Free Spice Blend

2 cups fresh raspberries

1 cup blackberries

⅔ cup unbleached all-purpose flour

¼ cup packed brown sugar

¼ cup trans fat–free light margarine or spread, chilled

Frozen yogurt (optional)

DIRECTIONS

Note: For each teaspoon of the NutriFit Certainly Cinnamon Salt Free Spice Blend you may substitute: ½ tsp. cinnamon, ¼ tsp. nutmeg, ⅛ tsp. ginger, and ⅛ tsp. cloves.

1 Preheat the oven to 375°F.

2 Peel and slice the peaches into 1¼-inch thick wedges. (If fresh peaches are unavailable you may use canned or frozen peach slices.) In a shallow, 1½- to 2-quart baking dish, combine the peaches, granulated sugar, lemon juice, and spice blend; mix lightly. Spread the berries over the peach mixture.

3 In a medium bowl, mix together the flour and brown sugar until well blended. Cut in the margarine and blend the mixture until it begins to cling together in lumps. Spoon over the berries.

4 Bake for about 30 minutes, or until bubbly. Let cool for at least 10 minutes; serve warm. Top with frozen yogurt (optional).

STORAGE INSTRUCTIONS

Refrigerate promptly; may be frozen.

NUTRIENT INFORMATION (serving size: 1 cup):
Calories: 126; Protein: 2 g; Carbohydrates: 30.5 g; Fat: 0.6 g; Fiber: 4.2 g

OTHER BENEFICIAL NUTRIENTS:
Excellent source of: vitamin A, vitamin C
Good source of: fiber

peanut butter and jelly sandwich

SERVINGS: 1

INGREDIENTS

1 Tbsp. reduced-fat, all-natural peanut butter

2 slices whole-wheat bread

1 tsp. low-sugar strawberry spread

DIRECTIONS

1 Spread the peanut butter on one slice of bread.

2 Spread the jelly on the other slice of bread.

3 Put the bread together into a sandwich.

STORAGE INSTRUCTIONS

Store at room temperature.

NUTRIENT INFORMATION (serving size: 1 sandwich):
Calories: 226; Protein: 9.3 g; Carbohydrates: 31.5 g; Fat: 8.4 g; Fiber: 4 g

OTHER BENEFICIAL NUTRIENTS:
Excellent source of: folacin
Good source of: iron, zinc, fiber

peanut butter–hot fudge dip

INGREDIENTS

½ cup unsweetened cocoa powder

¾ cup sugar

1 cup fat-free milk

½ cup fat-free evaporated milk

3 Tbsp. reduced-fat, all-natural peanut butter

2 tsp. vanilla extract

DIRECTIONS

1 Place the cocoa and sugar in a 1½-quart saucepan and mix well. Slowly whisk in the two types of milk. Cook over medium heat for 5 minutes, or just until the mixture comes to a boil, stirring constantly.

2 Reduce the heat to low, add the peanut butter, and cook and stir for 2 minutes, or until the peanut butter has melted. Remove the pan from the heat and stir in the vanilla.

3 Serve the dip warm, with cake or graham cracker squares, fresh strawberries, and/or chunks of banana, pineapple, apple, or pear.

STORAGE INSTRUCTIONS

Refrigerate promptly; do not freeze.

NUTRIENT INFORMATION (serving size: 2 Tbsp.):
Calories: 80; Protein: 2.5 g; Carbohydrates: 14.5 g; Fat: 1.4 g; Fiber: 1 g

OTHER BENEFICIAL NUTRIENTS:
Excellent source of: vitamin A

peanut butter wrap

INGREDIENTS

1⅛ cups reduced-fat, all-natural peanut butter

1 (12.3-oz) pkg. extra-firm, reduced fat tofu

2 pieces lavosh

2 apples, peeled, cored, and thinly sliced

DIRECTIONS

1 In a food processor, combine the peanut butter and tofu, and process until well mixed.

2 Spread each piece of lavosh lightly with the peanut butter mixture. Arrange apple slices evenly over the top. Roll and cut each lavosh roll into 6 even pieces. Serve immediately or wrap in plastic wrap and refrigerate until ready to eat.

STORAGE INSTRUCTIONS

Refrigerate promptly; do not freeze.

NUTRIENT INFORMATION (serving size: two 4-inch pieces):
Calories: 364; Protein: 20.4 g; Carbohydrates: 32.1 g; Fat: 17.9 g; Fiber: 2.6 g

OTHER BENEFICIAL NUTRIENTS:
Excellent source of: folacin
Good source of: fiber

peanut noodles and veggies

SERVINGS: 4

INGREDIENTS

7 Tbsp. water

¼ cup reduced-fat, all-natural creamy peanut butter

2 Tbsp. brown sugar

1 Tbsp. reduced-sodium soy sauce

2 Tbsp. rice vinegar

1½ tsp. peeled and minced fresh ginger

1 tsp. sesame oil

½ tsp. cornstarch

2 cloves garlic, minced

8 oz. dry udon noodles (Japanese wheat noodles)

1 cup carrots thinly sliced on the diagonal

½ cup canned water chestnuts, drained and thinly sliced

1 cup snow peas, ends and strings removed

½ cup asparagus, sliced on the diagonal

2 cups sliced bok choy

DIRECTIONS

1 In a small saucepan, combine the water, peanut butter, brown sugar, soy sauce, rice vinegar, ginger, sesame oil, cornstarch, and garlic; stir with a whisk until blended. Bring the mixture to a boil; cook for 1 minute, stirring constantly. Set aside.

2 Put the vegetables in a microwave-safe bowl and cook on high for 2 minutes or until crisp-tender.

3 Cook the noodles in boiling water for 8 minutes. Drain well. In a large bowl, combine the noodles, peanut sauce, and vegetables and toss well to coat.

STORAGE INSTRUCTIONS

Refrigerate promptly; do not freeze.

NUTRIENT INFORMATION (serving size: 2 cups):
Calories: 399; Protein: 14.7 g; Carbohydrates: 67.5 g; Fat: 9.5 g; Fiber: 7.9 g

OTHER BENEFICIAL NUTRIENTS:
Excellent source of: vitamin A, vitamin C, folacin, fiber
Good source of: iron, zinc

piña colada dip

SERVINGS: 6

INGREDIENTS

¼ cup Neufchâtel light cream cheese

6 oz. extra-firm, reduced-fat tofu

½ cup vanilla fat-free yogurt

½ small banana, peeled and mashed

2 Tbsp. frozen apple-juice concentrate

1 tsp. golden raisins

¼ tsp. NutriFit Certainly Cinnamon Salt Free Spice Blend

½ cup canned unsweetened pineapple slices

DIRECTIONS

Note: For each teaspoon of the NutriFit Certainly Cinnamon Salt Free Spice Blend you may substitute: ½ tsp. cinnamon, ¼ tsp. nutmeg, ⅛ tsp. ginger, and ⅛ tsp. cloves.

1 In a food processor, combine the Neufchâtel cheese and tofu and process until smooth. Add the yogurt, banana, and apple-juice concentrate. Pulse to blend just until smooth.

2 Mix in the raisins, spice blend, and pineapple by hand. Serve the mixture as a dip with various fruits on the side, or eat with a spoon.

STORAGE INSTRUCTIONS

Refrigerate promptly; do not freeze.

NUTRIENT INFORMATION (serving size: ¼ cup):
Calories: 67; Protein: 3.9 g; Carbohydrates: 12.5 g; Fat: 0.4 g; Fiber: 0.6 g

OTHER BENEFICIAL NUTRIENTS:
Good source of: vitamin C

pork chops with onions and apples

SERVINGS: 6

INGREDIENTS

Extra-virgin olive oil cooking spray

6 (5-oz.) boneless pork chops

1 tsp. NutriFit Calypso Salt Free Spice Blend

1 medium onion, sliced

1 medium apple, cut into wedges

1 tsp. cornstarch

½ cup reduced-sodium beef broth

DIRECTIONS

Note: For each teaspoon of the NutriFit Calypso Salt Free Spice Blend you may substitute: ½ tsp. ground chiles, ¼ tsp. ground cumin, ⅛ tsp. black pepper, and ⅛ tsp. garlic powder.

1 Heat a skillet over medium heat until hot. Coat with cooking spray. Season the chops with the spice blend. Add the pork chops and cook (in 2 batches) for about 10 minutes, until browned. Remove the chops from the pan; set aside.

2 Remove the pan from the heat and coat again with cooking spray. Add the onions and apple and cook over medium heat until tender-crisp. Remove from the pan; set aside.

3 In a small bowl, mix the cornstarch and the broth until smooth, and add the mixture to the skillet. Cook until the mixture boils and thickens, stirring constantly.

4 Return the chops and the onion mixture to the pan, cover, and cook over low heat for about 5 minutes, until the pork is no longer pink in the center.

STORAGE INSTRUCTIONS

Refrigerate promptly; may be frozen.

NUTRIENT INFORMATION (serving size: 1 chop):
Calories: 235; Protein: 31.2 g; Carbohydrates: 5.4 g; Fat: 9 g; Fiber: 0.8 g

OTHER BENEFICIAL NUTRIENTS:
Excellent source of: vitamin B$_6$, zinc
Good source of: vitamin A

pork kabobs

INGREDIENTS

1 lb. pork tenderloin, trimmed of fat

2 Tbsp. hickory marinade or barbecue sauce

½ red onion, cut into 1-inch pieces

DIRECTIONS

1 Rinse the pork well, dry it with paper towels, then cut into 1½-inch cubes. Place in a glass bowl, pour the marinade over the pork, and turn to coat evenly. Cover with plastic wrap and refrigerate for 20–30 minutes.

2 Prepare the kabobs by placing alternating cubes of pork and onions on bamboo skewers that have been soaked in water for 20 minutes.

3 Grill or broil the skewers for about 15–20 minutes, until the pork is thoroughly cooked.

STORAGE INSTRUCTIONS

Refrigerate promptly; may be frozen.

NUTRIENT INFORMATION (serving size: 2 kabobs):
Calories: 260; Protein: 42.7 g; Carbohydrates: 3.2 g; Fat: 7.3 g; Fiber: 0.2 g

OTHER BENEFICIAL NUTRIENTS:
Excellent source of: vitamin B_6, zinc
Good source of: iron

power snack mix

SERVINGS: 8

INGREDIENTS

1 cup Chex Mix

1 cup raisins

¾ cup roasted soy nuts

1 cup shredded-wheat cereal

1 cup small pretzels

DIRECTIONS

1 In a large bowl, combine all of the ingredients. Divide into ⅔-cup servings and bag each serving separately.

2 Store at room temperature, away from heat and light.

STORAGE INSTRUCTIONS

Store in a cool, dry place.

NUTRIENT INFORMATION (serving size: ⅔ cup):
Calories: 171; Protein: 7.1 g; Carbohydrates: 29.7 g; Fat: 3.5 g; Fiber: 2.7 g

OTHER BENEFICIAL NUTRIENTS:
Good source of: iron, fiber

quinoa super salad

INGREDIENTS

1 cup Italian green beans (fresh or frozen)

5 cups cooked quinoa (cooked and cooled according to package directions)

1 cup diced carrots

½ cup finely chopped Italian parsley

¼ cup sliced black olives

½ cup sunflower seed kernels

¼ cup reduced-sodium tamari

¼ cup lemon juice

1 Tbsp. extra-virgin olive oil

1 cup tomatoes, fresh or canned, peeled, seeded, and chopped

DIRECTIONS

1 Steam the green beans until crisp-tender, or, if using frozen, defrost and drain.

2 Place the quinoa in a large serving bowl. Add the carrots, parsley, olives, green beans, and sunflower seeds to the quinoa. Mix thoroughly.

3 Combine the tamari and lemon juice with the olive oil, pour over the quinoa, and toss well. Garnish with tomatoes.

STORAGE INSTRUCTIONS

Best eaten within two days; do not freeze.

NUTRIENT INFORMATION (serving size: 1 cup):
Calories: 288; Protein: 8.9 g; Carbohydrates: 50.2 g; Fat: 8.3 g; Fiber: 6.1 g

OTHER BENEFICIAL NUTRIENTS:
Excellent source of: vitamin A, vitamin C, folacin, fiber

raisin oatmeal cookies

YIELD: 3½ DOZEN

INGREDIENTS

¼ cup fat-free egg substitute

1 cup packed brown sugar

2 Tbsp. canola oil

¾ cup plain fat-free yogurt

2 tsp. vanilla extract

2 cups old-fashioned oats

1½ cups unbleached all-purpose flour

1½ tsp. baking soda

1½ tsp. NutriFit Certainly Cinnamon Salt Free Spice Blend

¼ tsp. salt

1 cup raisins

DIRECTIONS

Note: For each teaspoon of the NutriFit Certainly Cinnamon Salt Free Spice Blend you may substitute: ½ tsp. cinnamon, ¼ tsp. nutmeg, ⅛ tsp. ginger, and ⅛ tsp. cloves.

1 Preheat the oven to 350°F. Line two baking sheets with parchment paper, or lightly coat with cooking spray.

2 In a small bowl, beat the egg substitute, brown sugar, and oil with an electric mixer until smooth. Add the yogurt and vanilla and beat again. Add the oats, flour, baking soda, spice blend, and salt and beat until well mixed. Stir the raisins into the batter.

3 Drop the batter by rounded teaspoonfuls about 2 inches apart onto the prepared baking sheets. Bake for 10–12 minutes, or until the cookies are lightly browned. Cool on a wire rack.

STORAGE INSTRUCTIONS

Store at room temperature; may be frozen.

NUTRIENT INFORMATION (serving size: 1 cookie):
Calories: 118; Protein: 2.8 g; Carbohydrates: 30 g; Fat: 2 g; Fiber: 1.3 g

ratatouille

INGREDIENTS

2 tsp. olive oil

½ cup chopped onion

3 cloves garlic, minced

1 large red bell pepper, cut into
1-inch pieces

1 large green bell pepper, cut
into 1-inch pieces

1 medium eggplant, peeled and
cut into 1-inch pieces

2 small zucchini, cut into
¼-inch-thick slices

1 Tbsp. NutriFit Mediterranean
Salt Free Spice Blend

½ tsp. sugar

¼ tsp. salt

1 bay leaf

1½ cups reduced-sodium
canned diced tomatoes

DIRECTIONS

Note: For each teaspoon of the NutriFit Mediterranean Salt Free Spice Blend you may substitute: ¼ tsp. basil, ¼ tsp. oregano, ¼ tsp. garlic powder, and ¼ tsp. black pepper.

1 Heat a large saucepan; add the olive oil, onion, and garlic; sauté for 3 minutes, until the onions are limp.

2 Add the bell peppers, eggplant, zucchini, spice blend, sugar, salt, and bay leaf. Cook for 10 minutes, stirring occasionally.

3 Add the tomatoes; cover, reduce the heat, and cook for 10 minutes, or until the vegetables are tender. Remove the bay leaf before serving.

STORAGE INSTRUCTIONS

Refrigerate promptly; may be frozen.

NUTRIENT INFORMATION (serving size: 1½ cups):
Calories: 97; Protein: 2.7 g; Carbohydrates: 15.8 g; Fat: 3.3 g; Fiber: 6.2 g

OTHER BENEFICIAL NUTRIENTS:
Excellent source of: vitamin A, vitamin C, folacin, fiber
Good source of: vitamin B_6

roast beef

INGREDIENTS

1 lb. rump beef roast

1 Tbsp. onion soup and dip mix

¼ cup red wine

3 ears of corn

DIRECTIONS

1 Place the roast in a roasting pan. Rub the meat with the onion soup mix and pour the wine over the meat. Cover and refrigerate, if marinating, for up to two days. When ready to cook, remove the meat from the refrigerator and let it sit for 20 minutes to come to room temperature.

2 Preheat the oven to 350°F.

3 Roast the meat for 20–30 minutes, or until thoroughly cooked. The recommended internal temperature for rare meat that is considered safe for consumption is 145°F, which can be checked with a meat thermometer.

4 Clean and rinse the corn; steam for 7–10 minutes. Serve with a slice of roast beef.

STORAGE INSTRUCTIONS

Refrigerate promptly; may be frozen.

NUTRIENT INFORMATION (serving size: 4 oz., or a piece about the size of a deck of playing cards):
Calories: 334; Protein: 45.3 g; Carbohydrates: 15.8 g; Fat: 8.5 g; Fiber: 2.1 g

OTHER BENEFICIAL NUTRIENTS:
Excellent source of: vitamin B_6, zinc
Good source of: vitamin A, folacin, iron

roasted tomato soup

SERVINGS: 6

INGREDIENTS

Olive oil cooking spray

3 lb. ripe tomatoes, cored, seeded, and halved (8–10 medium-size)

1½ tsp. olive oil

1 cup coarsely chopped red onion

3 cloves garlic, minced

3 cups reduced-sodium vegetable broth

3 Tbsp. chopped basil

Salt and pepper to taste

DIRECTIONS

1 Preheat the broiler. Coat a baking sheet with cooking spray and place the tomatoes on it, cut side down. Broil the tomatoes for 10-12 minutes, or until the skins are blistered and blackened. Let cool, then slip off the skins.

2 Heat a medium-size saucepan, add the oil and the onions, and cook for 5 minutes. Add the garlic and cook for 2 minutes more, or until the onions are softened. In a food processor or a blender, combine the tomatoes and onions and process until smooth. Return the soup to the saucepan.

3 Add the vegetable broth and bring to a boil. Reduce the heat to low and simmer the soup for 5 minutes. Remove the pan from the heat and stir in the basil. Season the soup with salt and pepper.

STORAGE INSTRUCTIONS

Refrigerate promptly; may be frozen.

NUTRIENT INFORMATION (serving size: 1¼ cups):
Calories: 73; Protein: 2.4 g; Carbohydrates: 13.9 g; Fat: 1.9 g; Fiber: 3.1 g

OTHER BENEFICIAL NUTRIENTS:
Excellent source of: vitamin A, vitamin C, folacin
Good source of: vitamin B_6, fiber

roasted vegetables

SERVINGS: 3

INGREDIENTS

1 small butternut squash, peeled, seeded, and cut into 1-inch cubes (1 cup)

1 cup carrots peeled and cut into ½-inch rounds

1 cup cubed potato

1 cup peeled and cubed rutabaga

2 tsp. olive oil

2 tsp. NutriFit Calypso Salt Free Spice Blend

DIRECTIONS

Note: For each teaspoon of the NutriFit Calypso Salt Free Spice Blend you may substitute: ½ tsp. ground chiles, ¼ tsp. ground cumin, ⅛ tsp. black pepper, and ⅛ tsp. garlic powder.

1 Preheat the oven to 400°F.

2 Coat the vegetables with the olive oil, then sprinkle them with the spice blend. If you don't enjoy rutabagas, you may substitute parsnips or turnips.

3 Spread the vegetables out on a baking sheet. Bake for 30–40 minutes, until tender.

STORAGE INSTRUCTIONS

Refrigerate promptly; do not freeze.

NUTRIENT INFORMATION (serving size: 1¼ cups):
Calories: 175; Protein: 3.5 g; Carbohydrates: 35.3 g; Fat: 3.4 g; Fiber: 6.7 g

OTHER BENEFICIAL NUTRIENTS:
Excellent source of: vitamin A, vitamin C, vitamin B$_6$, folacin, fiber
Good source of: iron

rockin' moroccan sirloin roast

SERVINGS: 6

INGREDIENTS

2 lbs. rump beef roast

2 tsp. Rockin' Moroccan Salt Free Spice Blend

1 cup red wine

1 bay leaf

DIRECTIONS

Note: For each teaspoon of the NutriFit Rockin' Moroccan Salt Free Spice Blend you may substitute: ½ tsp. cumin, ⅛ tsp. thyme, ⅛ tsp. cayenne pepper, ⅛ tsp. turmeric, and ⅛ tsp. coriander.

1 Wash and cut the fat off the roast. Pat dry with paper towels.

2 Rub the roast on all sides with the spice blend. Let stand for 1 hour, covered, in the refrigerator (longer is fine).

3 When ready to cook the roast, remove from the refrigerator and sear the roast in a hot skillet on all sides. Put in a roasting pan, pour wine around it, and add the bay leaf.

4 Roast at 350°F for 20 minutes, cut to test, and finish roasting until the meat tests done at 145°F internal temperature. Let stand before slicing, to seal in the meat juices.

STORAGE INSTRUCTIONS

Refrigerate promptly; may be frozen.

NUTRIENT INFORMATION (serving size: 5 oz., or a piece about the size of an audio cassette tape):
Calories: 334; Protein: 45.3 g; Carbohydrates: 15.8 g; Fat: 8.5 g; Fiber: 2.1 g

OTHER BENEFICIAL NUTRIENTS:
Excellent source of: vitamin B$_6$, zinc
Good source of: vitamin A, folacin, iron

sautéed fish fillets with lime

SERVINGS: 3

INGREDIENTS

1⅓ lbs. (3 fillets) cod

3 Tbsp. whole-wheat flour

1 clove garlic, minced

1 Tbsp. lime juice

1 Tbsp. trans fat–free light margarine or spread, melted

⅓ cup dry white wine

1 Tbsp. extra-virgin olive oil

3 green onions, chopped

DIRECTIONS

1 Rinse the fish fillets and pat them dry with paper towels. Coat the fillets with the flour; set aside.

2 In a bowl, add the minced garlic, lime juice, and margarine to the wine.

3 Heat a skillet over medium-high heat. Add the oil and the fillets, and cook the fillets (do not overlap the fish) until golden on the bottom; turn over and cook about 1 minute more, until the fish flakes easily with a fork. Transfer the fish to a platter and keep warm.

4 Add the wine mixture to the pan and bring to a boil, scraping up cooked bits from the bottom of the pan, until the liquid is reduced by half. Reduce the heat to low, stir in the onions and cook for about 30 seconds. Pour the sauce over the fish.

STORAGE INSTRUCTIONS

Refrigerate promptly; do not freeze.

NUTRIENT INFORMATION (serving size: 6 oz., or a fillet about the size of the palm of your hand):
Calories: 229; Protein: 17 g; Carbohydrates: 11 g; Fiber: 10.33 g
Excellent source of: vitamin B_{12}, protein
Good source of: iron

scrambled eggs and onions

INGREDIENTS

1 tsp. extra-virgin olive oil

3 cups fat-free egg substitute

1 tsp. NutriFit Calypso Salt Free Spice Blend

3 green onions, finely chopped

DIRECTIONS

Note: For each teaspoon of the NutriFit Calypso Salt Free Spice Blend you may substitute: ½ tsp. ground chiles, ¼ tsp. ground cumin, ⅛ tsp. black pepper, and ⅛ tsp. garlic powder.

1 Heat a nonstick skillet until hot, then add the oil.

2 Add the egg substitute, spice blend, and green onions. Cook, stirring, until the eggs are set. Serve immediately.

STORAGE INSTRUCTIONS

Refrigerate promptly; do not freeze.

NUTRIENT INFORMATION (serving size: 1 cup):
Calories: 128; Protein: 24.2 g; Carbohydrates: 3.6 g; Fat: 0.6 g; Fiber: 0.2 g

OTHER BENEFICIAL NUTRIENTS:
Excellent source of: vitamin A

seafood fajitas

SERVINGS: 3

INGREDIENTS

8 oz. cod fillets

8 oz. shrimp, peeled and deveined

1 Tbsp. NutriFit Calypso Salt Free Spice Blend

1 tsp. extra-virgin olive oil

2 cloves garlic, sliced

½ red onion, peeled and sliced

1 green bell pepper, cut into ¼-inch wide strips

1 yellow bell pepper, cut into ¼-inch wide strips

1 red bell pepper, cut into ¼-inch strips

⅔ cup fresh salsa, medium-spicy

DIRECTIONS

Note: For each teaspoon of the NutriFit Calypso Salt Free Spice Blend you may substitute: ½ tsp. ground chiles, ¼ tsp. ground cumin, ⅛ tsp. black pepper, and ⅛ garlic powder.

1 Cut the cod into chunks. Season the fish and shrimp with the spice blend. Cover the seafood with plastic wrap and marinate, refrigerated, for 30 minutes.

2 Heat a medium skillet, add the oil, garlic, onion, and bell peppers and sauté over high heat for about 3 minutes.

3 Add the seafood and cook for 5 minutes, stirring constantly, then add the salsa and serve immediately with additional salsa and tortillas or rice on the side (optional).

STORAGE INSTRUCTIONS

Refrigerate promptly; may be frozen.

NUTRIENT INFORMATION (serving size: 6 oz.):
Calories: 358; Protein: 50.9 g; Carbohydrates: 16.8 g; Fat: 9.8 g; Fiber: 4.7 g

OTHER BENEFICIAL NUTRIENTS:
Excellent source of: vitamin A, vitamin C, vitamin B$_6$, folacin, zinc, fiber
Good source of: calcium, iron

shrimp salad

INGREDIENTS

1 Tbsp. pine nuts, toasted

6 oz. shrimp, cooked and butterflied

¼ cup sliced carrots

¼ cup chopped tomatoes

¼ cup sliced cucumber

1 tsp. NutriFit Garden Salt Free Spice Blend

2 cups field greens

¼ cup tangerine segments

Fat-free or low-fat vinaigrette dressing

DIRECTIONS

Note: For each tablespoon of the NutriFit Lemon Garden Salt Free Spice Blend you may substitute: 1½ tsp. basil, ½ tsp. marjoram, ½ tsp. dill weed, and ½ tsp. black pepper.

1 Toast the pine nuts in a dry skillet or oven (at 350°F) until fragrant and light brown; set aside to cool.

2 Wash the shrimp and pat dry with paper towels. Place the cooked shrimp in a bowl and add the carrots, tomato, and cucumber. Season with the spice blend.

3 Mound the field greens in the center of a serving platter and top with the shrimp mixture. Garnish with the tangerine segments and refrigerate until ready to serve.

4 Just before serving, top with the pine nuts and serve with your choice of fat-free or low-fat vinaigrette dressing.

STORAGE INSTRUCTIONS

Refrigerate for up to one day; do not freeze.

NUTRIENT INFORMATION (serving size: 3 cups):
Calories: 291; Protein: 41.1 g; Carbohydrates: 15.6 g; Fat: 7.4 g; Fiber: 4.1 g

OTHER BENEFICIAL NUTRIENTS:
Excellent source of: vitamin A, vitamin C, vitamin B_6, folacin, zinc
Good source of: calcium, iron, fiber

southwest chicken and veggie salad

SERVINGS: 8

INGREDIENTS

Canola oil cooking spray

8 (4-oz.) boneless, skinless chicken breasts

Salt to taste

1 tsp. ground cumin

½ tsp. coarsely ground pepper

2 cloves garlic, finely minced

1½ lb. zucchini, unpeeled and cut into ¼-inch slices

1 cup finely chopped onion

2 small jalapeño or serrano peppers, seeded and chopped (optional)

1 lb. fresh tomatoes, peeled and cored

1 lb. frozen white corn kernels

12 cups shredded romaine lettuce

DIRECTIONS

1 Heat a large skillet and coat with cooking spray. Add the chicken, sprinkle with salt, and cook for 5 minutes on each side, or until lightly browned.

2 Add the cumin, pepper, and garlic, and cook for about 10 minutes, stirring occasionally. Add the zucchini, onion, hot peppers (optional), and tomatoes. Cover; do not add other liquid (as the mixture stews it will accumulate quite a bit of liquid). Cook for about 20 minutes.

3 Add the frozen corn and salt to taste. Uncover and cook for 15 minutes longer.

4 Cool, then serve over bed of shredded salad greens.

STORAGE INSTRUCTIONS

Refrigerate promptly; do not freeze.

NUTRIENT INFORMATION (serving size: 1 breast):
Calories: 336; Protein: 57.8 g; Carbohydrates: 17.4 g; Fat: 3.6 g; Fiber: 3.5 g

OTHER BENEFICIAL NUTRIENTS:
Excellent source of: vitamin A, vitamin C, vitamin B_6, folacin
Good source of: iron, zinc, fiber

spanish omelet

SERVINGS: 2

INGREDIENTS

4 egg whites

¼ cup water

½ tsp. NutriFit Calypso
Salt Free Spice Blend

1 cup fat-free egg substitute

Canola oil cooking spray

¼ cup chopped green bell
pepper

¼ cup chopped tomato

1 Tbsp. minced onion

½ cup grated reduced-fat
cheddar cheese

DIRECTIONS

Note: For each teaspoon of the NutriFit Calypso Salt Free Spice Blend you may substitute: ½ tsp. ground chiles, ¼ tsp. cumin, ⅛ tsp. black pepper, and ⅛ tsp. garlic powder.

1 In a bowl, beat the egg whites until bubbly. Add the water and spice blend and beat until thick.

2 In a separate bowl, beat the egg substitute. Fold the egg whites into the egg substitute.

3 Heat a nonstick skillet. When hot, coat with cooking spray and pour in half of the egg mixture. Reduce the heat and cook until the bottom is browned. Add half of the vegetables and fold the omelet over. Top with half the cheese and cook until cheese is melted.

4 Remove the omelet from the pan and repeat the process with the remaining ingredients.

STORAGE INSTRUCTIONS

Refrigerate promptly; do not freeze.

NUTRIENT INFORMATION (serving size: 1 omelet):
Calories: 134; Protein: 19.6 g; Carbohydrates: 6.7 g; Fat: 2.9 g; Fiber: 0.9 g

OTHER BENEFICIAL NUTRIENTS:
Excellent source of: vitamin A, vitamin C, calcium

spiced baked apples with walnuts

INGREDIENTS

1 Tbsp. chopped walnuts

⅓ cup apple juice

⅓ cup dry white wine

⅓ cup water

2 Tbsp. finely grated orange peel

4 medium-size apples

¼ tsp. cinnamon

1 Tbsp. raisins

DIRECTIONS

1 Preheat the oven to 375°F. Toast the walnuts until fragrant and golden brown; set aside.

2 In a small saucepan, simmer the apple juice, wine, and water for 10 minutes over low heat. Add the orange zest; set aside.

3 Core and peel the apples halfway down from the stem end. Place in a small nonreactive baking pan just large enough for the apples and reserved apple liquid. Generously sprinkle the apples with the cinnamon. Fill each apple center with raisins.

4 Bake for about 25–30 minutes, until the apples are tender but still hold their shape, basting with the pan juices every 10 minutes.

5 Serve the apples warm with 1 tablespoon of the pan juices spooned into the cored center. Top each serving with chopped walnuts.

STORAGE INSTRUCTIONS

Refrigerate promptly; do not freeze.

NUTRIENT INFORMATION (serving size: 1 apple):
Calories: 128; Protein: 0.9 g; Carbohydrates: 26.9 g; Fat: 1.6 g; Fiber: 4.3 g

OTHER BENEFICIAL NUTRIENTS:
Excellent source of: vitamin C
Good source of: vitamin A, vitamin B_6, fiber

spinach

INGREDIENTS

½ tsp. olive oil

2 Tbsp. chopped onion

¼ clove garlic, chopped (optional)

1 cup frozen chopped spinach

¼ tsp. NutriFit Lemon Garden Salt Free Spice Blend

DIRECTIONS

Note: For each teaspoon of the NutriFit Lemon Garden Salt Free Spice Blend you may substitute: ¼ tsp. basil, ¼ tsp. marjoram, ¼ tsp. black pepper, and ¼ tsp. dill weed.

1 Heat a nonstick skillet and add the olive oil. Then add the onions and sauté the onions until golden brown. Add the garlic (optional).

2 Add the spinach and spice blend.

3 Cover and cook until the spinach is heated through. Serve warm.

STORAGE INSTRUCTIONS

Refrigerate promptly; may be frozen.

NUTRIENT INFORMATION (serving size: 1 cup):
Calories: 116; Protein: 12.6 g; Carbohydrates: 24.7 g; Fat: 5.1 g; Fiber: 12.3 g

OTHER BENEFICIAL NUTRIENTS:
Excellent source of: vitamin A, vitamin C, folacin, calcium, zinc, fiber
Good source of: vitamin B_6, iron

spinach and chive dip

SERVINGS: 8

INGREDIENTS

1 lb. frozen chopped spinach

1 tsp. finely chopped chives

1 tsp. NutriFit Lemon Garden Salt Free Spice Blend

⅓ cup fat-free mayonnaise

⅓ cup fat-free sour cream

⅓ cup plain fat-free yogurt

1 Tbsp. dried dill weed

DIRECTIONS

Note: For each teaspoon of the NutriFit Lemon Garden Salt Free Spice Blend you may substitute: ¼ tsp. basil, ¼ tsp. marjoram, ¼ tsp. black pepper, and ¼ tsp. dill weed.

1 Defrost the spinach in the microwave oven or a sauté pan; drain well.

2 In a food processor, combine all of the ingredients. Pulse with short bursts to blend, being careful not to overmix. Taste for seasoning.

3 Chill until ready to serve.

STORAGE INSTRUCTIONS

Refrigerate promptly; do not freeze. Refrigerated, the dip will stay fresh for up to three days.

NUTRIENT INFORMATION (serving size: ¼ cup):
Calories: 43; Protein: 2.9 g; Carbohydrates: 6.7 g; Fat: 0 g; Fiber: 1.8 g

OTHER BENEFICIAL NUTRIENTS:
Excellent source of: vitamin A

spinach pilaf

SERVINGS: 8

INGREDIENTS

1 Tbsp. extra-virgin olive oil

1 cup chopped onion

2 cups uncooked brown basmati rice, washed and drained

3 cups water

2 Tbsp. NutriFit Lemon Garden Salt Free Spice Blend

¼ cup lemon juice

1½ lbs. frozen chopped spinach

DIRECTIONS

Note: For each tablespoon of the NutriFit Lemon Garden Salt Free Spice Blend you may substitute: 1½ tsp. basil, ½ tsp. marjoram, ½ tsp. dill weed, and ½ tsp. black pepper.

1 Heat a large sauté pan; add the oil and the onion. Sauté over medium heat until soft, stirring well. Add the washed and drained rice to the onion, and cook for 5 minutes, stirring.

2 Add the water, spice blend, and lemon juice; bring to a boil. When boiling, add the spinach, stir well, and cover tightly with the lid. Reduce the heat and simmer over low heat for 15 minutes.

3 Remove from the heat, leave tightly covered, and let stand for 5–10 minutes before serving. Also good served cold.

STORAGE INSTRUCTIONS

Refrigerate promptly; may be frozen.

NUTRIENT INFORMATION (serving size: ½ cup):
Calories: 108; Protein: 2.9 g; Carbohydrates: 21 g; Fat: 1 g; Fiber: 1.6 g

OTHER BENEFICIAL NUTRIENTS:
Good source of: iron, vitamin C

spinach salad with honey dijon dressing

SERVINGS: 6

INGREDIENTS

1 Tbsp. honey

2 Tbsp. balsamic vinegar

1 Tbsp. chopped Italian parsley

2 Tbsp. Dijon mustard

½ tsp. black pepper

4 Tbsp. reduced-sodium vegetable broth

1 Tbsp. water

1 Tbsp. canola oil

12 cups spinach leaves, coarsely chopped

2 cups sliced mushrooms

2 slices whole-wheat bread, cubed and toasted

DIRECTIONS

1 In a small glass bowl, heat the honey in a microwave oven until it liquefies. In a food processor, combine the honey, vinegar, parsley, mustard, black pepper, vegetable broth, and water, and process until smooth.

2 With the motor running, drizzle in oil until the dressing thickens and is well combined.

3 Serve over spinach greens, topped with mushrooms and croutons.

STORAGE INSTRUCTIONS

Refrigerate promptly; do not freeze. Refrigerated, the dressing will remain fresh for about two weeks.

NUTRIENT INFORMATION (serving size: 2 cups):
Calories: 49; Protein: 2.5 g; Carbohydrates: 7.2 g; Fat: 1.7 g; Fiber: 2 g

OTHER BENEFICIAL NUTRIENTS:
Excellent source of: vitamin A, vitamin C, folacin
Good source of: iron

spinach, cheese, and mushroom bake

SERVINGS: 6

INGREDIENTS

Canola oil cooking spray

3 Tbsp. dry white wine

4 cups sliced mushrooms
(about 12 oz.)

4 chopped green onions

1 tsp. NutriFit Lemon Garden
Salt Free Spice Blend

1½ lb. frozen spinach, defrosted
and well drained

½ cup dry bread crumbs

2 cups fat-free cottage cheese,
rinsed and drained

6 egg whites

DIRECTIONS

Note: For each teaspoon of the NutriFit Lemon Garden Salt Free Spice Blend you may substitute: ¼ tsp. basil, ¼ tsp. marjoram, ¼ tsp. black pepper, and ¼ tsp. dill weed.

1 Preheat the oven to 350°F. Lightly spray a 9x13-inch baking pan.

2 In a nonstick skillet, bring the wine to a boil. Add the mushrooms and green onions and cook until just tender. Add the spice blend and spinach (chop the spinach coarsely, if the leaves are large). Stir well, then transfer the mixture to a mixing bowl.

3 Mix in the bread crumbs and the drained cottage cheese.

4 Beat the egg whites until stiff and fold them gently into the spinach mixture. Pour the mixture into the prepared baking dish.

5 Bake, uncovered, for 30 minutes, or until firm. Let stand for 10 minutes before cutting.

STORAGE INSTRUCTIONS

Refrigerate promptly; do not freeze.

NUTRIENT INFORMATION (serving size: two 3-inch squares):
Calories: 286; Protein: 40.1 g; Carbohydrates: 30.9 g; Fat: 1.3 g; Fiber: 7.7 g

OTHER BENEFICIAL NUTRIENTS:
Excellent source of: vitamin A, vitamin C, vitamin B_6, folacin, calcium, fiber
Good source of: iron, zinc

spinach, tofu, and brown rice stir-fry

SERVINGS: 4

INGREDIENTS

1½ tsp. extra-virgin olive oil

1 cup chopped onion

2 cloves garlic, minced

1 (12.3-oz.) pkg. extra-firm, reduced-fat tofu, cut into cubes

1½ tsp. reduced-sodium soy sauce

2 tsp. NutriFit Mediterranean Salt Free Spice Blend

½ cup reduced-sodium V8 juice

1 cup spinach leaves, coarsely chopped

Dash Tabasco sauce

2 cups cooked brown rice

DIRECTIONS

Note: For each teaspoon of the NutriFit Mediterranean Salt Free Spice Blend you may substitute: ¼ tsp. basil, ¼ tsp. oregano, ¼ tsp. garlic powder, and ¼ tsp. black pepper.

1 Heat a nonstick skillet. Add the oil and sauté the onion and garlic for 3–5 minutes, stirring constantly.

2 Add the tofu, soy sauce, and spice blend; brown the tofu slightly.

3 Add the juice, spinach, and Tabasco, and cook for 5 minutes more.

4 Spoon the mixture over the hot rice.

STORAGE INSTRUCTIONS

Refrigerate promptly; may be frozen.

NUTRIENT INFORMATION (serving size: 2 cups):
Calories: 422; Protein: 25.4 g; Carbohydrates: 67.3 g; Fat: 6.8 g; Fiber: 11 g

OTHER BENEFICIAL NUTRIENTS:
Excellent source of: vitamin A, vitamin C, vitamin B$_6$, folacin, calcium, zinc, fiber
Good source of: iron

spinach, tomato, and red-onion salad

SERVINGS: 4

INGREDIENTS

5 cups spinach leaves, coarsely chopped

3 medium tomatoes, cut into ¼-inch slices

2 small red onions, halved lengthwise and thinly sliced

1½ Tbsp. balsamic vinegar

2 Tbsp. water

½ tsp. white pepper

2 Tbsp. orange juice

½ Tbsp. extra-virgin olive oil

1 Tbsp. chopped parsley

DIRECTIONS

1 Arrange the spinach on a platter or in a large, shallow bowl. Arrange the tomatoes over the spinach, and then the onions over the tomatoes.

2 In a small bowl, whisk together the vinegar, water, white pepper, and orange juice until thoroughly blended. Whisking continuously, incorporate the oil into the dressing mixture.

3 The dressing can be refrigerated at this point, or you may pour the dressing over the vegetables, garnish with parsley, and serve.

STORAGE INSTRUCTIONS

Refrigerate promptly; do not freeze.

NUTRIENT INFORMATION (serving size: 1¼ cups):
Calories: 61; Protein: 3.1 g; Carbohydrates: 9.3 g; Fat: 2.3 g; Fiber: 3.3 g

OTHER BENEFICIAL NUTRIENTS:
Excellent source of: vitamin A, vitamin C, folacin
Good source of: vitamin B_6, iron, fiber

steel-cut oats

SERVINGS: 1

INGREDIENTS

¾ cup water

⅓ cup steel-cut oats

1 tsp. brown sugar (optional)

DIRECTIONS

1 Boil the water and add the oats gradually.

2 Reduce the heat and cook for 8–10 minutes, stirring occasionally. Add sugar (optional).

3 Let stand; serve when desired consistency is reached.

STORAGE INSTRUCTIONS

Refrigerate promptly; do not freeze.

NUTRIENT INFORMATION (serving size: 1 cup):
Calories: 290; Protein: 12.2 g; Carbohydrates: 50.6 g; Fat: 4.7 g; Fiber: 8 g

OTHER BENEFICIAL NUTRIENTS:
Excellent source of: fiber
Good source of: vitamin A, folacin, iron, zinc

strawberries italiano

INGREDIENTS

1 qt. fresh strawberries

3 Tbsp. balsamic vinegar

4 Tbsp. sugar

⅓ cup pine nuts

Pinch ground cloves

1 pt. vanilla reduced-fat
frozen yogurt

DIRECTIONS

1 Wash the strawberries, remove the hulls, and slice. Place in a bowl. Mix the vinegar and 3 Tbsp. of the sugar. Pour over the berries. Let stand 30 minutes.

2 In a heavy, small skillet, toast the pine nuts with the remaining sugar and the cloves over medium-low heat, stirring constantly. Cook until the pine nuts are golden and the sugar has melted.

3 Scoop the yogurt into four bowls. Add the strawberries. Garnish with pine nuts.

STORAGE INSTRUCTIONS

Refrigerate promptly; do not freeze.

NUTRIENT INFORMATION (serving size: 1 cup):
Calories: 135; Protein: 4.8 g; Carbohydrates: 22.7 g; Fat: 3.8 g; Fiber: 1.7 g

OTHER BENEFICIAL NUTRIENTS:
Excellent source of: vitamin C
Good source of: folacin, calcium

stuffed portobello mushrooms

SERVINGS: 1

INGREDIENTS

Extra-virgin olive oil cooking spray

¼ cup finely chopped onion

1 clove garlic, minced

1½ cups frozen chopped spinach

1 tsp. NutriFit Mediterranean Salt Free Spice Blend

1½ oz. soy taco product

2 extra-large portobello mushrooms

2 oz. soy cheese, shredded

DIRECTIONS

Note: For each teaspoon of the NutriFit Mediterranean Salt Free Spice Blend you may substitute: ¼ tsp. basil, ¼ tsp. oregano, ¼ tsp. garlic powder, and ¼ tsp. black pepper.

1 Preheat the oven to 375°F.

2 Heat a sauté pan over medium heat, coat with cooking spray, and sauté the onion and the garlic until softened. Add the spinach, spice blend, and the soy taco meat. Cook for 10 minutes, or until the mixture is soft.

3 Stuff the mushroom caps with the spinach mixture, dividing evenly, and top with soy cheese.

3 Bake for 20–25 minutes, until cheese is melted and lightly browned.

STORAGE INSTRUCTIONS

Refrigerate promptly; may be frozen.

NUTRIENT INFORMATION (serving size: 2 mushrooms):
Calories: 329; Protein: 31.1 g; Carbohydrates: 21.3 g; Fat: 12.4 g; Fiber: 14.1 g

OTHER BENEFICIAL NUTRIENTS:
Excellent source of: vitamin A, calcium, fiber
Good source of: iron

stuffed squash with cheese

INGREDIENTS

2 medium-size acorn squash

1 Tbsp. olive oil

1 Tbsp. minced garlic

1 cup peeled and diced eggplant

1 cup diced red bell pepper

2 cups cooked brown rice

2 tsp. NutriFit Mediterranean Salt Free Spice Blend

¼ cup chopped parsley

1 Tbsp. balsamic vinegar

Pinch salt

¾ cup grated reduced-fat mozzarella cheese

DIRECTIONS

Note: For each teaspoon of the NutriFit Mediterranean Salt Free Spice Blend you may substitute: ¼ tsp. basil, ¼ tsp. oregano, ¼ tsp. garlic powder, and ¼ tsp. black pepper.

1 Preheat the oven to 375°F.

2 Using a large, heavy knife, carefully halve the squash lengthwise. Place the halves cut side down on a foil-lined baking sheet and bake for 20 minutes, or until the flesh is barely tender. Leave the oven set at 375°F.

3 Let the squash cool slightly, then remove and discard the seeds and stringy membranes. Using a teaspoon, scoop out and reserve the flesh, leaving a ¼-inch-thick shell and being careful not to pierce the skin; set aside the flesh and hollowed-out squash.

4 For the stuffing, heat the olive oil in a medium-size skillet over medium heat. Add the garlic and sauté for 15 seconds, then add the eggplant and sauté for 2–3 minutes, or until the eggplant begins to soften. Add the bell pepper and continue cooking for 2 minutes, stirring occasionally. Add the reserved squash flesh, rice, spice blend, parsley, vinegar, and salt, and stir to combine thoroughly.

5 Divide the mixture among the squash shells, top with the mozzarella, and bake for 10–15 minutes, or until the filling is heated through.

STORAGE INSTRUCTIONS

Refrigerate promptly; do not freeze.

NUTRIENT INFORMATION
(serving size: ½ filled squash):
Calories: 311; Protein: 11.8 g; Carbohydrates: 51.3 g; Fat: 8.4 g; Fiber: 9.8 g

OTHER BENEFICIAL NUTRIENTS:
Excellent source of: vitamin A, vitamin C, vitamin B$_6$, folacin, calcium, fiber
Good source of: iron, zinc

swedish muesli

SERVINGS: 1

INGREDIENTS

¾ cup plain fat-free yogurt

½ cup chopped apple (do not peel)

¼ cup muesli cereal

DIRECTIONS

1 In a bowl, blend the yogurt and chopped apple together.

2 Top the yogurt mixture with muesli cereal.

STORAGE INSTRUCTIONS

Refrigerate promptly; do not freeze.

NUTRIENT INFORMATION (serving size: 1½ cups):
Calories: 181; Protein: 11.1 g; Carbohydrates: 34.5 g; Fat: 0.5 g; Fiber: 3.1 g

OTHER BENEFICIAL NUTRIENTS:
Excellent source of: calcium
Good source of: folacin, zinc, fiber

sweet potato curry with lentils

INGREDIENTS

1 tsp. canola oil

1 large yam or sweet potato, peeled and cut into ½-inch dice (1 cup)

½ cup chopped onion

¼ tsp. black pepper

1 clove garlic, finely chopped

1 jalapeño pepper, seeded and finely chopped

½ tsp. peeled and grated fresh ginger

1 medium butternut squash, peeled, seeded, and cut into 1-inch chunks (1 cup)

1 cup vegetable broth

½ tsp. garam masala (optional)

½ cup cooked lentils

1 Tbsp. yogurt (optional)

DIRECTIONS

1 Heat a nonstick skillet, add the oil, and sauté the sweet potato over medium heat for 5 minutes, turning occasionally. Remove with a slotted spoon. Add the onion and cook for 5 minutes, or until transparent, stirring occasionally. Add the pepper, garlic, jalapeño pepper, and ginger and cook, stirring, for 1 minute.

2 Meanwhile, bring the butternut squash to a boil in a pan of water, then simmer until almost cooked. Drain and add to the skillet, along with half of the vegetable broth and the garam masala (optional). Stir to combine, bring to a simmer, and cover. Reduce the heat and simmer gently for 20 minutes, adding a little more stock if the curry looks too dry. Add the lentils during last 10 minutes of cooking.

3 If desired, stir in 1 Tbsp. yogurt, and serve with rice.

STORAGE INSTRUCTIONS

Best eaten within two days; do not freeze.

NUTRIENT INFORMATION (serving size: 1⅓ cups):
Calories: 278; Protein: 11.5 g; Carbohydrates: 54.5 g; Fat: 3 g; Fiber: 14.2 g

OTHER BENEFICIAL NUTRIENTS:
Excellent source of: vitamin A, vitamin C, vitamin B_6, folacin, fiber
Good source of: calcium, iron, zinc

thai basil chicken

INGREDIENTS

1 Tbsp. reduced-sodium soy sauce

¼ cup reduced-sodium chicken broth

¼ cup dry sherry

1 tsp. grated lime peel

½ cup chopped basil

1 Tbsp. peeled and chopped fresh ginger

2 tsp. cornstarch

1 lb. boneless, skinless chicken breasts

3 cloves garlic, minced

1 large onion, halved lengthwise and thinly sliced

2 fresh red chiles, seeded and chopped

1 Tbsp. canola oil

2 cups chopped green cabbage

DIRECTIONS

1 In a large bowl, combine the soy sauce, broth, sherry, lime peel, basil, ginger, and cornstarch. Cut the chicken into 2-inch strips and add to the marinade; cover and refrigerate for 30 minutes.

2 In a wok or large skillet, stir-fry the garlic, onion, and chiles in the oil over low heat for 2 minutes. Using a slotted spoon, add the chicken to the wok, reserving the marinade. Stir-fry for 4 minutes. Add the reserved marinade to the wok; cook for another 2–3 minutes, until the chicken is done and the sauce thickens. Serve on a bed of chopped cabbage.

STORAGE INSTRUCTIONS

Refrigerate promptly; may be frozen.

NUTRIENT INFORMATION (serving size: 5 oz. chicken breast):
Calories: 204; Protein: 39.6 g; Carbohydrates: 4.3 g; Fat: 2.2 g; Fiber: 0.6 g

OTHER BENEFICIAL NUTRIENTS:
Excellent source of: vitamin A, vitamin C, vitamin B_6
Good source of: zinc

tofu chili

INGREDIENTS

2 tsp. extra-virgin olive oil

1 clove garlic, finely chopped

2 medium-size green bell peppers, seeded and chopped

1 cup chopped onion

4 tsp. NutriFit Calypso Salt Free Spice Blend

¼ tsp. red pepper flakes (optional)

1 (28-oz.) can reduced-sodium crushed tomatoes

½ tsp. salt

8 oz. extra-firm, reduced-fat tofu, crumbled

1 (15-oz.) can reduced-sodium cannellini beans, drained

1 (15-oz.) can reduced-sodium garbanzo beans, drained

DIRECTIONS

Note: For each teaspoon of the NutriFit Calypso Salt Free Spice Blend you may substitute: ½ tsp. ground chiles, ¼ tsp. cumin, ⅛ tsp. black pepper, and ⅛ tsp. garlic powder.

1 Heat a heavy saucepan over medium heat; add the oil, garlic, green pepper, and onion, and sauté until tender but not browned.

2 Sprinkle with the spice blend and pepper flakes (optional). Cook, stirring, for 1 minute.

3 Add the tomatoes, salt, and tofu. Bring to a boil and simmer for 15 minutes. Add the beans. Let stand for several hours or refrigerate overnight (to intensify the flavors) before reheating to serve.

STORAGE INSTRUCTIONS

Refrigerate promptly; may be frozen.

NUTRIENT INFORMATION (serving size: 1 cup):
Calories: 187; Protein: 15 g; Carbohydrates: 30.9 g; Fat: 2.8 g; Fiber: 10 g

OTHER BENEFICIAL NUTRIENTS:
Excellent source of: vitamin A, vitamin C, vitamin B_6, fiber

tofu hoisin with vegetables and walnuts

SERVINGS: 4

INGREDIENTS

1 (12.3-oz.) pkg. extra-firm, reduced-fat tofu

1 tsp. sesame oil

1 Tbsp. reduced-sodium tamari

⅓ cup hoisin sauce

2 Tbsp. sake

1 tsp. canola oil

6 cloves garlic, minced

⅛ tsp. red pepper flakes (optional)

2 medium-size red bell peppers, cut into strips

3 cups broccoli flowerets

4 Tbsp. chopped walnuts

⅓ cup water

DIRECTIONS

1 Cut the tofu into 1-inch cubes. Season with ½ tsp. of the sesame oil and the tamari. In a cup, combine the hoisin sauce, sake, and remaining sesame oil, and set aside.

2 Heat a wok or large skillet over high heat until hot, but not smoking. Add the canola oil. Make sure the tofu is patted very dry to prevent sticking and add the tofu to the wok. Stir-fry until lightly golden. Transfer the tofu to a platter and reduce the heat to medium-high.

3 Add the garlic and crushed red pepper flakes (optional) and cook for 1 minute. Stir in the red bell pepper, broccoli, and walnuts and toss to coat with the garlic. Pour in the water, toss the vegetables, then cover the pan. Cook for 5 minutes, or until vegetables are tender but crunchy.

4 Stir in the tofu, then pour in the sauce mixture. Stir-fry for 1 minute, or until the sauce coats everything and is thickened. May be served with steamed brown rice.

STORAGE INSTRUCTIONS

Refrigerate promptly; do not freeze.

NUTRIENT INFORMATION (serving size: 1 cup):
Calories: 378; Protein: 14.6 g; Carbohydrates: 40.9 g; Fat: 9.5 g; Fiber: 4.1 g

OTHER BENEFICIAL NUTRIENTS:
Excellent source of: vitamin A, vitamin C, vitamin B_6, folacin
Good source of: calcium, iron, fiber

tomato tuna salad

INGREDIENTS

1 (6.5-oz.) can solid white tuna packed in water, drained

¾ Tbsp. fresh lemon juice

½ Tbsp. fat-free mayonnaise

1 green onion, ends trimmed, diced

¼ cup chopped bell pepper

¼ cup diced celery

Dash salt-free lemon pepper seasoning

2 large tomatoes

4 large lettuce leaves

DIRECTIONS

1 Empty the tuna into a colander. Separate the tuna into big chunks with a fork, then rinse it gently and drain it well. Place the tuna in a small mixing bowl.

2 Add the lemon juice, mayonnaise, green onions, bell pepper, celery, and seasoning. Stir well, breaking up any large chunks of tuna.

3 Core the tomatoes and cut into quarters, making sure you do not cut all the way through the base of the the tomato. Open the tomatoes up like a flower, put on a bed of lettuce leaves, and fill with the tuna mixture, dividing evenly.

STORAGE INSTRUCTIONS

Refrigerate promptly; do not freeze.

NUTRIENT INFORMATION (serving size: 3 oz. tuna, or ⅔ cup):
Calories: 161; Protein: 23.3 g; Carbohydrates: 10.1 g; Fat: 3.2 g; Fiber: 2.2 g

OTHER BENEFICIAL NUTRIENTS:
Excellent source of: vitamin A, vitamin C, vitamin B_6
Good source of: folacin, iron

tomato, mozzarella, and basil salad

SERVINGS: 4

INGREDIENTS

2 Tbsp. red-wine vinegar

1 clove garlic, minced

⅛ tsp. salt

¼ tsp. dry mustard

Dash fresh ground black pepper

1 Tbsp. extra-virgin olive oil

4 Italian plum tomatoes

6 oz. fat-free mozzarella cheese

9 basil leaves, packed, washed, dried, and stemmed

¼ cup finely chopped Italian parsley

DIRECTIONS

1 For the dressing, combine the vinegar, garlic, salt, mustard, and pepper in a small bowl. Add the oil in slow, steady stream, whisking until the oil is thoroughly blended.

2 Slice the tomatoes and cheese into ¼-inch-thick slices. Trim the cheese slices to the size of the tomato slices.

3 Place the tomato and cheese slices in a large shallow bowl or glass baking dish. Pour the dressing over the slices. Marinate, covered, in the refrigerator for at least 30 minutes or up to 3 hours, turning the slices occasionally.

4 Layer the basil leaves with the largest leaf on the bottom, then roll up jelly-roll fashion. Slice the basil roll into ¼-inch-thick slices; separate into strips.

5 Arrange the tomato and cheese slices alternately on a serving platter or four individual salad plates. Sprinkle with basil strips, drizzle with the remaining dressing, and top with parsley.

STORAGE INSTRUCTIONS

Refrigerate promptly; do not freeze.

NUTRIENT INFORMATION (serving size: 1 cup):
Calories: 248; Protein: 28.1 g; Carbohydrates: 18.4 g; Fat: 7.8 g; Fiber: 3.2 g

OTHER BENEFICIAL NUTRIENTS:
Excellent source of: vitamin A, vitamin C, folacin, calcium
Good source of: vitamin B_6, iron, fiber

tomato, potato, and eggplant gratin

SERVINGS: 6

INGREDIENTS

Canola oil cooking spray

1 large eggplant, unpeeled, cut crosswise into ¼-inch-thick slices

2 Tbsp. olive oil

1 large onion, thinly sliced

1 medium red bell pepper, seeded and finely chopped

1 (28-oz.) can reduced-sodium chopped tomatoes, undrained

3 cloves garlic, minced or pressed

½ tsp. thyme

¼ tsp. sugar

5 large russet potatoes

Chopped parsley (optional)

DIRECTIONS

1 Preheat the broiler. Coat a large, shallow baking dish with cooking spray. Arrange the eggplant slices in a single layer in the pan; coat with cooking spray. Broil about 4 inches below the heat for 6–8 minutes, until well browned. Turn the eggplant slices over, coat the other sides with cooking spray, and broil 5–6 more minutes, until browned. Set aside.

2 Heat the oil in a large skillet over medium heat. Add the onion and bell pepper. Cook for 8–10 minutes, until the vegetables are soft but not browned, stirring often. Stir in the tomatoes, garlic, thyme, and sugar. Cook for 3 minutes, stirring often, then remove from the heat.

3 Preheat the oven to 375°F. Peel and thinly slice the potatoes. Spray a large, shallow baking dish with cooking spray. Spread a third of the potatoes in the prepared dish. Top with half the eggplant, then half the tomato sauce. Cover with half the remaining potatoes and add the remaining eggplant and tomato sauce. Top with the remaining potatoes.

4 Bake for 1–1¼ hours, until the potatoes are lightly browned on top and tender when pierced. Sprinkle with chopped parsley (optional).

STORAGE INSTRUCTIONS

Refrigerate promptly; may be frozen.

NUTRIENT INFORMATION
(serving size: 1½ cups):
Calories: 277; Protein: 7 g;
Carbohydrates: 55 g; Fat: 5 g;
Fiber: 8.6 g

OTHER BENEFICIAL NUTRIENTS:
Excellent source of: vitamin A, vitamin C, vitamin B$_6$, folacin, fiber
Good source of: iron

turkey burger

INGREDIENTS

1 lb. lean ground turkey

½ cup fat-free egg substitute

¼ cup quick-cooking rolled oats

1 tsp. NutriFit Calypso Salt Free Spice Blend

1 tsp. extra-virgin olive oil

DIRECTIONS

Note: For each teaspoon of the NutriFit Calypso Salt Free Spice Blend you may substitute: ½ tsp. ground chiles, ¼ tsp. cumin, ⅛ tsp. black pepper, and ⅛ tsp. garlic powder.

1 In a medium-size bowl, mix the turkey, egg substitute, oats, and spice blend. Shape the turkey mixture into four patties, each about ½ inch thick.

2 Heat a wide, nonstick skillet. Add the olive oil, then the turkey patties. Cook for 8–10 minutes, turning once, until the patties are lightly browned on both sides and the juices run clear when a knife is inserted in the center.

STORAGE INSTRUCTIONS

Refrigerate promptly; may be frozen.

NUTRIENT INFORMATION (serving size: one 4-oz. burger):
Calories: 200; Protein: 22 g; Carbohydrates: 4 g; Fat: 10 g; Fiber: 2 g

OTHER BENEFICIAL NUTRIENTS:
Good source of: zinc, iron

turkey salad

INGREDIENTS

Canola oil cooking spray

1 lb. turkey breast

1 tsp. NutriFit Calypso Salt Free
Spice Blend

1 tsp. extra-virgin olive oil

½ cup diced celery

3 green onions, chopped

½ cup fat-free mayonnaise

¼ tsp. paprika

DIRECTIONS

Note: For each teaspoon of the NutriFit Calypso Salt Free Spice Blend you may substitute: ½ tsp. ground chiles, ¼ tsp. cumin, ⅛ tsp. black pepper, and ⅛ tsp garlic powder.

1 Preheat the oven to 350°F, or coat a nonstick skillet with cooking spray.

2 Rinse the turkey and pat it dry. Cut the turkey into cubes and season with the spice blend and olive oil.

3 Cook the turkey in a baking dish in the oven, covered, or the skillet, covered, about 12–15 minutes, until thoroughly cooked. Let cool. This can be done up to 2 days in advance.

4 In a bowl, combine the diced celery, onion, mayonnaise, and paprika. Add the cubed turkey and mix together. Refrigerate until ready to serve.

STORAGE INSTRUCTIONS

Refrigerate promptly; do not freeze.

NUTRIENT INFORMATION (serving size: ¾ cup):
Calories: 151; Protein: 28.2 g; Carbohydrates: 5.2 g; Fat: 0.8 g; Fiber: 0.5 g

OTHER BENEFICIAL NUTRIENTS:
Excellent source of: vitamin A, vitamin B_6
Good source of: iron, zinc

turkey wrap

SERVINGS: 1

INGREDIENTS

3 oz. turkey breast, cooked

½ piece whole-wheat lavosh

¼ cup chopped tomato

¾ cup shredded romaine lettuce

1 tsp. fat-free Italian dressing

DIRECTIONS

1 Slice the cooked turkey breast into strips.

2 Place the turkey in the center of the lavosh square. Place the tomatoes and lettuce on top of the turkey, and fold the lavosh bread and roll.

3 Serve with the dressing on the side.

STORAGE INSTRUCTIONS

Refrigerate promptly; do not freeze.

NUTRIENT INFORMATION (serving size: 1 wrap):
Calories: 198; Protein: 13 g; Carbohydrates: 33.2 g; Fat: 0.9 g; Fiber: 1.2 g

OTHER BENEFICIAL NUTRIENTS:
Excellent source of: vitamin A, vitamin C, folacin
Good source of: vitamin B_6

vegan wrap

SERVINGS: 1

INGREDIENTS

1 oz. soy cheese

1 (6-in.) piece lavosh

¼ cup thinly sliced celery

¾ cup shredded romaine
lettuce

1 small tomato, thinly sliced

½ avocado, diced

DIRECTIONS

1 Cut the soy cheese into matchsticks.

2 In the center of the piece of lavosh, place the vegetables
and soy cheese.

3 Fold up the sides of the lavosh and skewer with a toothpick.

STORAGE INSTRUCTIONS

Refrigerate promptly; do not freeze.

BODY AFTER BABY

NUTRIENT INFORMATION (serving size: 1 wrap):
Calories: 410; Protein: 14.8 g; Carbohydrates: 44.7 g; Fat: 20.1 g; Fiber: 6.7 g

OTHER BENEFICIAL NUTRIENTS:
Excellent source of: vitamin A, vitamin C, vitamin B$_6$, folacin,
calcium, fiber
Good source of: iron

vegetable barley soup

SERVINGS: 4

INGREDIENTS

Extra-virgin olive oil
cooking spray

½ cup diced onion

½ cup diced carrot

½ cup diced celery

1 cup sliced mushrooms

½ cup pearl barley

⅔ cup dried green split peas

¼ tsp. salt

¼ tsp. black pepper

6 cups water

DIRECTIONS

1 Heat a 3-quart saucepan and coat with cooking spray.
Sauté the onions, carrots, and celery for 5–10 minutes.
Add the mushrooms and sauté for 1 minute more.

2 Rinse the barley and peas in a colander; drain. Add to the
pan with the vegetables and season with salt and pepper.

3 Add the water and bring to a boil. Reduce the heat, cover,
and cook for about 30 minutes, until the barley and peas
are tender.

STORAGE INSTRUCTIONS

Refrigerate promptly; may be frozen.

NUTRIENT INFORMATION (serving size: 1 cup):
Calories: 214; Protein: 10.7 g; Carbohydrates: 50.3 g; Fat: 1.2 g;
Fiber: 14.4 g

OTHER BENEFICIAL NUTRIENTS:
Excellent source of: vitamin A, vitamin C, fiber
Good source of: folacin, iron

vegetable-stuffed turkey roll

SERVINGS: 3

INGREDIENTS

1 lb. fresh ground turkey

¼ cup dry whole-wheat bread crumbs, or 1 slice whole-wheat bread, crumbled

¼ cup fat-free egg substitute

¼ cup chopped Italian parsley

¼ tsp. black pepper

½ tsp. thyme

1 cup chopped fresh broccoli

½ cup chopped mushrooms

¼ cup chopped red bell pepper

1 clove garlic, minced

2 Tbsp. catsup

1 tsp. prepared mustard

DIRECTIONS

1 Preheat the oven to 350°F. Line a nonstick loaf pan with waxed paper or spray with nonstick cooking spray; set aside.

2 In a large mixing bowl, combine the turkey, bread crumbs, egg substitute, parsley, pepper, and thyme; mix well. Pat the mixture out to an 8-inch square on a large piece of plastic wrap; set aside.

3 In a small microwave-safe bowl, combine the broccoli, mushrooms, bell pepper, and garlic. Cook in the microwave for 2–3 minutes, or until the vegetables are tender but crisp (or you may sauté them in a nonstick skillet.)

4 Spoon the vegetable mixture to within 1 inch of the edges of the turkey mixture. Roll the turkey mixture into a loaf by lifting the plastic wrap until the turkey begins to roll tightly, peeling away the wrap as you roll. Place it in the prepared pan.

5 Mix the catsup with the mustard, and spread evenly over the top. Bake for 45 minutes, or until the roll is cooked through.

STORAGE INSTRUCTIONS

Refrigerate promptly; may be frozen.

NUTRIENT INFORMATION (serving size: two 2-inch slices):
Calories: 277; Protein: 34 g; Carbohydrates: 13 g; Fat: 10 g; Fiber: 1.5 g

OTHER BENEFICIAL NUTRIENTS:
Excellent source of: vitamin C, protein, folate, fiber
Good source of: vitamin B_{12}

vegetarian bean enchiladas

INGREDIENTS

8 oz. dried pinto beans, soaked overnight, or 2 cups canned, drained

1 tsp. NutriFit Calypso Salt Free Spice Blend

1 cup shredded reduced-fat cheddar cheese

Vegetable oil cooking spray

2 tsp. olive oil

½ cup chopped onion

2 cloves garlic, minced

1 cup chunky salsa

¼ cup no-salt-added tomato paste

¼ tsp. seeded and finely chopped jalapeño pepper

¼ cup chopped cilantro

1 tsp. red-wine vinegar

12 (6-inch) corn tortillas

NUTRIENT INFORMATION
(serving size: 2 enchiladas):
Calories: 366; Protein: 18.2 g;
Carbohydrates: 60.4 g; Fat: 5.9 g;
Fiber: 10.6 g

OTHER BENEFICIAL NUTRIENTS:
Excellent source of: vitamin A, calcium, fiber

DIRECTIONS

Note: For each teaspoon of the NutriFit Calypso Salt Free Spice Blend you may substitute: ½ tsp. ground chiles, ¼ tsp. cumin, ⅛ tsp. black pepper, and ⅛ tsp. garlic powder.

1 If using dried beans, drain the beans and place in a 2-quart saucepan. Add cold water to cover. Bring to a boil over high heat. Reduce the heat to low, partially cover the pan, and simmer for 1½–2 hours, or until tender.

2 Drain the beans and transfer to a large bowl. Stir in the spice blend and ¾ cup of the cheddar cheese; set aside.

3 Preheat the oven to 350°F. Coat two 9x13-inch baking dishes with cooking spray; set aside.

4 In a large, nonstick skillet warm the oil over medium heat. Add the chopped onions and garlic, stirring frequently until tender. Stir in the salsa, tomato paste, peppers, and cilantro; bring to a boil. Then reduce the heat to low and simmer until the sauce thickens slightly. Stir in the vinegar.

5 Briefly dip each tortilla into the sauce to coat and soften. Place 2 rounded tablespoons of the bean filling on each tortilla; roll to enclose the filling. Place, seam side down, in one of the prepared baking dishes. Repeat to use the remaining tortillas. Spoon the remaining sauce evenly over the enchiladas. Sprinkle with the remaining ¼ cup cheese.

6 Cover the pans with foil and bake for 15–20 minutes, or until the cheese has melted and the sauce is bubbly.

STORAGE INSTRUCTIONS

Refrigerate promptly; may be frozen.

vegetarian enchilada casserole

INGREDIENTS

Canola oil cooking spray

1 cup enchilada sauce

8 (6-inch) corn tortillas

2 cups cooked brown rice

1½ cups fresh tomato salsa

2 cups vegetarian refried beans

1 cup chopped green onions

2 tsp. NutriFit Calypso Salt Free Spice Blend

1 cup shredded reduced-fat cheddar cheese

1 cup shredded reduced-fat Monterey Jack cheese

DIRECTIONS

Note: For each teaspoon of the NutriFit Calypso Salt Free Spice Blend you may substitute: ½ tsp. ground chiles, ¼ tsp. cumin, ⅛ tsp. black pepper, and ⅛ tsp. garlic powder.

1 Preheat the oven to 350°F. Coat a 9x13-inch baking dish with cooking spray. Pour just enough of the enchilada sauce into the prepared dish to lightly coat the bottom. Put one layer of tortillas in the dish, overlapping them slightly if necessary.

2 In a bowl, mix the cooked brown rice with ½ cup of the salsa.

3 Combine the refried beans, green onions, and spice blend. Spread the bean mixture over the tortillas, then add a thin layer of the rice. Spoon some of the salsa over the casserole, then top with a sprinkling of each type of cheese. Repeat the layers until all ingredients are used up, reserving a small amount of cheese for the top.

4 Pour the remaining enchilada sauce over the casserole and top with the reserved cheese. Bake, uncovered, for about 20 minutes, until the cheese is melted and the casserole is heated through. Cut into squares to serve.

STORAGE INSTRUCTIONS

Refrigerate promptly; may be frozen.

NUTRIENT INFORMATION (serving size: 2-inch square):
Calories: 204; Protein: 11.9 g; Carbohydrates: 32.7 g; Fat: 3.6 g; Fiber: 2.5 g

OTHER BENEFICIAL NUTRIENTS:
Excellent source of: vitamin A, calcium
Good source of: vitamin C, vitamin B$_6$, folacin, zinc, fiber

warm pineapple rings

SERVINGS: 4

INGREDIENTS

1 tsp. trans fat–free light margarine or spread

½ tsp. brown sugar

8 slices fresh pineapple, or canned pineapple

¼ tsp. cinnamon

DIRECTIONS

1 Heat a skillet or griddle over medium heat. Melt the margarine, then add the sugar and cook until bubbling.

2 Add the pineapple slices and heat on both sides, spraying with additional cooking spray as needed. Sprinkle the pineapple with cinnamon.

STORAGE INSTRUCTIONS

Refrigerate promptly; do not freeze.

NUTRIENT INFORMATION (serving size: 2 slices):
Calories: 107; Protein: 0.8 g; Carbohydrates: 26.4 g; Fat: 0 g; Fiber: 1.2 g

OTHER BENEFICIAL NUTRIENTS:
Excellent source of: vitamin C

wild berry smoothie

SERVINGS: 3½

INGREDIENTS

3 cups unsweetened apple juice

1 (12.3-oz.) pkg. extra-firm, reduced-fat tofu

½ cup frozen unsweetened strawberries

½ cup frozen unsweetened blueberries

1 small banana

DIRECTIONS

1 Pour the juice into a blender. Add the tofu and fruit and process until smooth.

2 May be refrigerated for up to four days. The mixture will separate when standing, but can be processed again to homogenize.

STORAGE INSTRUCTIONS

Refrigerate promptly; may be frozen.

BODY AFTER BABY

NUTRIENT INFORMATION (serving size: 8 oz.):
Calories: 288; Protein: 17 g; Carbohydrates: 48 g; Fat: 0.6 g; Fiber: 3.7 g

OTHER BENEFICIAL NUTRIENTS:
Excellent source of: vitamin C, vitamin B_6
Good source of: vitamin A, folacin, calcium, iron, fiber

wild rice pilaf

INGREDIENTS

1 cup uncooked wild rice

2½ cups water

½ cup dry white wine

¼ tsp. salt

Canola oil cooking spray

⅓ cup sliced green onion

½ tsp. thyme

¼ tsp. black pepper

¼ cup pine nuts, toasted

2 Tbsp. minced parsley

DIRECTIONS

1 Rinse the wild rice in three changes of hot water; drain. In a saucepan, combine the 2½ cups water, wine, and salt; bring to a boil. Add the rice; cover, reduce the heat, and simmer for 1 hour. Drain; set aside.

2 Coat a large nonstick skillet with cooking spray; place over medium-high heat until hot. Add the green onions and sauté until tender. Stir in the rice, thyme, and pepper.

3 Top with the toasted pine nuts and parsley.

STORAGE INSTRUCTIONS

Refrigerate promptly; may be frozen.

NUTRIENT INFORMATION (serving size: ½ cup):
Calories: 151; Protein: 5.8 g; Carbohydrates: 20.8 g; Fat: 3.4 g; Fiber: 2 g

OTHER BENEFICIAL NUTRIENTS:
Good source of: vitamin A

yogurt cucumber sauce

SERVINGS: 4

INGREDIENTS

½ cup peeled and finely chopped cucumber

½ tsp. salt

1 cup plain fat-free yogurt

1 green onion, minced

1 clove garlic, minced

2 Tbsp. chopped mint

DIRECTIONS

1 Place the cucumber in a colander, mix with the salt, and let drain for 20 minutes. Rinse the cucumbers with cold water and pat dry with paper towels.

2 In a medium-size bowl, combine the cucumber, yogurt, green onion, garlic, and mint; mix well with a whisk. Chill the sauce for at least 20 minutes, to develop the flavors. Serve the sauce with toasted pita-bread wedges or lavosh strips.

STORAGE INSTRUCTIONS

Refrigerate promptly; do not freeze.

BODY AFTER BABY

NUTRIENT INFORMATION (serving size: ½ cup):
Calories: 80; Protein: 7 g; Carbohydrates: 12 g; Fat: 0.2 g; Fiber: 0.4 g

OTHER BENEFICIAL NUTRIENTS:
Excellent source of: vitamin A, folacin, calcium
Good source of: vitamin C, iron, zinc

yogurt spread

INGREDIENTS

2 cups plain reduced-fat yogurt

DIRECTIONS

1 Line a sieve with a coffee filter or cheesecloth; suspend the sieve over a deep bowl. Place the yogurt in the filter and refrigerate for several hours or overnight, to allow the whey to drip out.

2 When the yogurt has thickened to the texture of soft cream cheese, scrape the yogurt away from the filter, transferring it to a resealable plastic container. Discard the liquid in the bowl.

3 Refrigerate for up to one week, discarding any accumulated liquid before using.

4 Can be used as a base for dips or dressings. Add your favorite fresh herbs or seasonings just before using.

STORAGE INSTRUCTIONS

Refrigerate promptly; do not freeze.

NUTRIENT INFORMATION (serving size: ¼ cup):
Calories: 48; Protein: 4 g; Carbohydrates: 5.3 g; Fat: 1.2 g; Fiber: 0 g

OTHER BENEFICIAL NUTRIENTS:
Good source of: vitamin A, calcium

zucchini with mushrooms

SERVINGS: 6

INGREDIENTS

½ cup reduced-sodium
chicken broth

4 cups coarsely diced zucchini

3 cloves garlic, minced

1 Tbsp. hot mustard

2 cups whole button
mushrooms

1 medium-size green bell
pepper, cut into ¼-inch strips

1 Tbsp. finely chopped
green onion

½ tsp. white pepper

DIRECTIONS

1 Preheat a wok or deep skillet and add the chicken broth.
Bring to a boil, and add the zucchini, garlic, and hot mustard, stirring once.

2 Add the mushrooms and green pepper and cook, stirring
for 1 minute. Reduce the heat to medium and cook for
2 minutes.

3 Add the green onion and white pepper. Increase the heat
to high and stir for a few seconds. Serve hot.

STORAGE INSTRUCTIONS

Refrigerate promptly; do not freeze.

NUTRIENT INFORMATION (serving size: ⅔ cup):
Calories: 43; Protein: 4 g; Carbohydrates: 6.1 g; Fat: 1.8 g; Fiber: 1.8 g

OTHER BENEFICIAL NUTRIENTS:
Excellent source of: vitamin A
Good source of: vitamin C, vitamin B_6, folacin

shopping lists

A Note About Shopping

Be sure to read labels when you're shopping. Key words and health claims on these labels are defined in accordance with government regulations, and claims on them like "fat-free" and "cholesterol-free" can only be used if a food actually meets legal standards. The food label titled Nutrition Facts is easy to read and trustworthy, and by law it should be on every packaged food product you buy. An important new addition to the labels is the line that reads "Trans Fats" and tells us how much of these potentially harmful hydrogenated oils are in the product. If there is zero to one-half gram of trans fats per serving, you aren't putting your body at risk.

The Nutrition Facts label lists nutrients that should be limited in a healthy diet—saturated fat, trans fat, and sodium—and also indicates the percentage of the Daily Value ("%DV") of healthful fiber, vitamins A and C, calcium, and iron that each serving of the product provides. Be sure to read the Nutrition Facts label on products you purchase, and be aware of the specified "Servings" in each package, since it may contain more than one.

There are many key words for each nutrient on food labels, and this language is

Start Here

Nutrition Facts

Serving Size 1 cup (228g)
Servings Per Container 2

Amount Per Serving

Calories 250	Calories from Fat 110

	% Daily Value*
Total Fat 12g	18%
Saturated Fat 3g	15%
Trans Fat 1.5g	
Cholesterol 30mg	10%
Sodium 470mg	20%
Total Carbohydrate 31g	10%
Dietary Fiber 0g	0%
Sugars 5g	
Protein 5g	

Vitamin A	4%
Vitamin C	2%
Calcium	20%
Iron	4%

Limit These Fats

Get Enough of
These Nutrients

Footnote

* Percent Daily Values are based on a 2,000 calorie diet.
Your Daily Values may be higher or lower depending on
your calorie needs:

	Calories:	2,000	2,500
Total Fat	Less than	65g	80g
Sat Fat	Less than	20g	25g
Cholesterol	Less than	300mg	300mg
Sodium	Less than	2,400mg	2,400mg
Total Carbohydrate		300g	375g
Dietary Fiber		25g	30g

Quick Guide to % DV
5% or less is low
20% or more is high

also governed by FDA guidelines. Remember that all of the terms are based on standard serving sizes.

- Fat-free = less than 0.5 grams fat per serving
- Very low and low-fat = less than 3 grams fat per serving
- Reduced-fat or less fat = product has 25% less fat than the standard version of the same food
- Low saturated fat = product has 1 gram or less saturated fat per serving
- Low-calorie = product has 40 calories or less per serving
- Low-cholesterol = product has 20 milligrams or less and 2 grams or less saturated fat
- Low-sodium = product has 140 milligrams or less per serving
- Excellent source of fiber = greater than 5 grams per serving

By law, all food labels must list ingredients in descending order by weight. The ingredient that weighs the most will be listed first, and the ingredient present in the least amount is listed last. For example, if you see sugar listed first, it is a sure sign that the product is full of sugar.

When reading ingredient lists, do not be misled. Sugars come in a variety of guises. Watch for ingredients such as honey, molasses, corn syrup, dextrose, fructose, galactose, glucose, lactose, maltose, and sucrose—these are all sugars.

When checking sodium content, be aware of other ingredients besides salt that contain sodium, including: baking powder, baking soda, and any additive that contains the word sodium (disodium, monosodium, and trisodium).

Don't be misled by words such as vegetable oils, as these are not necessarily beneficial. Palm and coconut oils are high in saturated fat. Look for products that contain unsaturated fats, such as corn, olive, peanut, safflower, soybean, olive, and canola oils.

THE SHOPPING LISTS

Quantities in the following shopping lists reflect the ingredients necessary to make the full number of servings of each recipe in the *Body After Baby* plan. If you're making just one serving, adjust the quantities you buy accordingly.

Shopping List for a Well-Stocked Kitchen

Keep these items on hand for quick, easy cooking while you're on the *Body After Baby* plan. You'll use all of these ingredients in the recipes on the plan. You probably have many of these items in your pantry already, but if not, here's a list. It's a great list to use anytime, whether you're on the *Body After Baby* plan or not. I've included the quantities that you will need to make all the recipes in the 30-day plan.

This list is designed to help create diverse and delicious flavors every day. But it's also very flexible to suit your personal taste and your budget. If you have a single favorite vinegar, maybe you don't want four. If you already have rolled oats on hand, you may choose to eliminate the steel-cut oats from your pantry. In this shopping list I'm offering you the full range of tastes—you can pick and choose according to your personal favorites. That said, I encourage you to try new things that may quickly become new favorites!

Recommended Pantry Additions: Non-Vegetarian

NUTS/SEEDS/DRIED FRUIT/ NUT BUTTERS/JAM/HONEY

Almonds, whole

Almonds, slivered (optional)

Currants, 4 oz.

Dates, unsweetened diced

Dried apple chips, 1 small pkg.

Dried cranberries, 1 cup

Dried fruits, mixed (such as apples, apricots, pears, and prunes) 2½ cups (1 lb.)

Dried pineapple, 1 cup

Figs, 2 cups dried

Honey, 1 small jar

Macadamia nuts

Peanut butter, 2 jars all-natural, reduced-fat

Peanuts

Pecans

Pine nuts

Pistachios

Preserves, 1 small jar all-fruit strawberry

Pumpkin seeds

Raisins, 1 lb. black or golden

Sesame seeds, 2 oz.

Soy nuts, 1 cup roasted

Sunflower seed kernels, 1 small pkg.

Walnuts

CANNED PRODUCTS—VEGETABLES/FRUITS/ SOUPS/BROTH/BEANS/TUNA

Applesauce, 1 (8-oz.) jar unsweetened

Apricot halves, 1 (16-oz.) can unsweetened, juice-packed

Artichoke hearts, 1 (16-oz.) can

Baby corn, 1 (1-lb.) can

Baby food prunes

Beans, 2 cans black

Beans, garbanzo, 2 (1-lb.) cans reduced-sodium

Beans, 1 (14-oz) can vegetarian refried

Beans, 1 (15-oz.) can white

Broth, 1 qt. beef (Choose lowest in sodium.)

Broth, 1 pint chicken (Choose lowest in sodium.)

Broth, 1 qt. vegetable (Choose lowest in sodium.)

Capers, 1 small jar

Mandarin orange segments, 1 (4-oz.) can

Miso soup, 1 can low-sodium instant

Olives, 1 (8-oz) can black (or green)

Olives, 1 small jar green

Onion soup and dip mix, 1 pkg. (Choose lowest in sodium.)

Pear halves, 1 (15-oz.) can, juice-packed

Pickles, 1 jar dill

Pineapple chunks in juice, 1 can

Pineapple slices in juice, 1 can

Ramen soup, 1 small pkg., any flavor (Discard the seasoning packet.)

Tomatoes, 2 (28-oz.) cans crushed

Tomatoes, 2 (28-oz.) cans plum/Italian

Tomatoes, 1 (8-oz) can stewed

Tuna, 1 (6.5-oz) can solid white, packed in water

Condiments (Oil/Vinegar/ Ready-to-Use Sauces)

Barbecue sauce, 1 small bottle hickory-flavored

Canola oil

Canola oil cooking spray

Catsup

Enchilada sauce, 1 (14-oz.) can

Hoisin sauce, 1 (4-oz.) jar

Marinara sauce, 2 cans/bottles (Choose lowest in sodium; no more than 4 g fat per serving.)

Mayonnaise, 1 qt. fat-free

Mesquite marinade, 1 small bottle

Mustard, Dijon

Mustard, 1 small jar hot (sometimes found in Asian food section)

Olive oil cooking spray, extra-virgin

Olive oil, extra-virgin

Salad dressing, lower-fat (less than 5 gm fat per serving)

Sesame oil, 1 small bottle toasted

Sesame tahini sauce, 1 small jar

Soy sauce, reduced-sodium

Tabasco sauce, 1 small bottle

Teriyaki sauce/marinade, 1 bottle (Choose lowest in sodium.)

Tomato sauce, 2 (8-oz.) cans no-salt-added

Vinegar, 1 small bottle apple-cider

Vinegar, 1 large bottle balsamic

Vinegar, 1 small bottle red-wine

Vinegar, rice, seasoned

Vinegar, 1 small bottle tarragon

Vinegar, 1 small bottle white

Worcestershire sauce, 1 small bottle

Worcestershire sauce, 1 small bottle white-wine

Spices and Herbs

Arrowroot (If unavailable, you may substitute cornstarch.)

Basil, dried

Bay leaves

Black pepper

Cayenne pepper

Chinese five-spice powder

Cream of tartar

Cumin

Dill weed

Lemon-pepper seasoning, salt-free

Meat tenderizer (optional)

Mint, dried

Mustard, dry

NutriFit Salt Free Spice Blends: Certainly Cinnamon, Mediterranean, Lemon Garden, Rockin' Moroccan, Calypso (**Note:** If not using NutriFit Spice Blends, then stock up on cinnamon and salt-free chili powder.)

Oregano, dried

Paprika

Sea salt

Sun-dried tomatoes, 1 small pkg.

Thyme

Turmeric

White pepper

CEREALS/BREADS/SNACK MIXES

Bagels, small whole-wheat

Biscotti

Bread, whole-wheat cinnamon

Bread, whole-grain

Bread, round (for phase 2 artichoke dip)

Breadcrumbs

buns, 1 pkg. sprouted-wheat burger-style (or cracked wheat)

Cereal, 1 small box 100% bran flakes

Cereal, 1 small box Grape-Nuts

Cereal, 1 small box muesli

Cereal, 1 lb. multigrain hot either oat-based or another blend of grains

Cereal, 1 small box oat flakes

Cereal, 1 small box unsweetened bite-sized shredded-wheat squares

Chex Mix, 1 small pkg. reduced-fat

Cookies, low-fat

Crackers, animal

Crackers, graham low-fat

Crackers, whole grain

English muffins, whole-wheat

Fig bars

Gingersnaps

Lavosh, 1 (1-lb.) pkg. whole-wheat (If unavailable, use whole-wheat tortillas.)

Oatmeal, instant

Oats, 1 carton (generally 1 lb. 14-oz.) steel-cut

Oats, 1 carton (generally 1 lb. 14-oz.) old-fashioned rolled

Oats, 1 carton (generally 1 lb. 14-oz.) quick-cooking rolled

Pita bread, whole wheat

Popcorn, air-popped

Pretzels, peanut-butter-filled

Pretzels, 1 (8-oz.) bag whole-grain (look for whole-wheat or oat bran)

Rice cakes, whole-grain

Rolls, whole-wheat

Tortillas, 6-inch corn

Tortillas, 10-inch whole-wheat flour

Vanilla wafers

Wheat germ

DRY GRAINS/LEGUMES

Barley, 1 lb. pearl

Cornmeal, 1 small box yellow

Couscous, 1 box whole-wheat

Green peas, 1 lb. dried split

Lentils, 1 (1-lb.) pkg. brown

Lentils, 1 (1-lb.) pkg. red (If red are unavailable, use brown.)

Noodles, 1 lb. lasagna

Pasta, whole-wheat linguine

Pasta, 1 lb. whole-wheat penne

Pasta, 1 lb. whole-wheat spaghetti

Pasta, whole-wheat vermicelli

Rice, 1 lb. brown basmati or other long-grain brown

Rice noodles

Rice, wild

BAKING SUPPLIES

Almond extract, 1 small bottle

Baking powder, 1 small can

Baking soda, 1 small box

Chocolate chips, 1 pkg. mini

Chocolate chips, 1 small pkg. semisweet

Cocoa powder, 1 small can unsweetened

Cornstarch, 1 box

Flour, cake

Flour, 5 lbs. whole-wheat

Flour, 5 lbs. unbleached all-purpose (preferably King Arthur brand White Whole Wheat, available via the Internet at the King Arthur Baking Company online store)

Maple syrup, 1 small bottle reduced-calorie/reduced-sugar

Milk, 3 (12-oz.) cans fat-free evaporated

Sugar, 1 lb. brown

Sugar, 1 lb. granulated

Sugar, 1 lb. powdered (or confectioners')

Vanilla extract, 1 small bottle

ALCOHOL FOR COOKING

Cooking sherry

Cooking wine, dry red

Cooking wine, dry white

FROZEN VEGETABLES/FROZEN FRUIT/FROZEN FRUIT JUICE/VEGETARIAN MEAT SUBSTITUTES

Apple-juice concentrate, 1 (12-oz) can frozen

Blueberries, 1 (1-lb.) pkg. frozen unsweetened

Cherries, 1 (1-lb.) pkg. frozen unsweetened pitted

Corn kernels, 2 (1-lb.) pkgs. frozen

Green peas, 1 (1-lb.) pkg. frozen

Strawberries, 1 (1-lb.) pkg. frozen unsweetened

Spinach, 1 (1-lb.) pkg. frozen chopped

Spinach, 1 (1-lb.) pkg. frozen leaf

Vegetables, frozen mixed

Vegetarian sausage links (usually 8- to 10-oz. box), 1 small pkg. frozen

Veggie burgers (usually 1-lb. box), 1 small pkg. frozen

Waffles, 1 pkg. frozen whole-grain

CANNED/BOTTLED JUICES

Apple juice, 1 (64-oz.) can unsweetened

Lemon juice, 1 small bottle reconstituted

Lime juice, 1 small bottle (or add fresh limes for each stage)

Orange juice, 1 pint fresh, preferably calcium-fortified

Pineapple juice, 1 (6-oz.) can unsweetened

V8 juice, 1 (6-oz.) can reduced-sodium

DAIRY

Margarine or spread, 1 (4-oz.) container trans fat–free light

Parmesan cheese, grated, reduced-fat or fat-free

Sour cream, 1 pint fat-free or low-fat

Soy milk, 1 cup light vanilla

Tofu, 2 (12-oz. to 1-lb.) pkgs. boxed firm (preferably light or reduced-fat, or use fresh tofu.)

Phase 1 Shopping List

DAIRY

Cheese, 1 (8-oz.) pkg. cheddar, reduced-fat, brick or shredded

Cheese, 1 (4-oz.) container cream cheese, fat-free or reduced-fat (Neufchâtel)

Cheese, 1 (4-oz.) container feta, reduced-fat

Cheese, light (Baby Bonbel Light or similar), 1 small pkg.

Cheese, 1 (8-oz.) pkg. mozzarella, reduced-fat or part-skim milk

Cheese, 1 (2–4-oz.) pkg. provolone

Cheese, 1 (8-oz.) container ricotta, fat-free or part-skim milk

Cheese, string, reduced-fat, 1 small pkg.

Cottage cheese, 1 pint fat-free or low-fat

Egg substitute, liquid

Eggs, 1 dozen (Store in coldest part of refrigerator in original packaging.)

Ice cream, reduced-fat chocolate, 1 pint

Milk, 2 gallons fat-free

Yogurt, 5 (8-oz.) containers fat-free vanilla

MEATS, POULTRY, AND SEAFOOD

Chicken, 4 lbs. boneless, skinless breasts (Buy fresh and freeze, or buy frozen.)

Cod, 2½ lb. fillets (Buy fresh and freeze, or buy frozen.)

Ham, 3 oz.

Pork, ¼ lb. center-cut loin chops, or other lean cut (Buy fresh and freeze, or buy frozen.)

Ravioli, chicken-stuffed, 1 (9-oz.) pkg.

Roast beef, 4 oz. deli

Salmon, 1 lb. (Buy fresh and freeze, or buy frozen.)

Shrimp, ½ lb. cooked (Buy fresh and freeze, or buy frozen.)

Shrimp, ½ lb. raw, peeled, and deveined (Buy fresh and freeze, or buy frozen.)

Turkey, 3 lb. plus 3 oz. cooked boneless, skinless breasts (Buy fresh and freeze, or buy frozen.)

Turkey, 2 links sausages (Buy fresh and freeze, or buy frozen.)

FRESH PRODUCE

Apples, 7 Granny Smith or other (Store in plastic bag in produce bin of refrigerator.)

Bananas, 6 (Store in pantry, away from heat, light, and tomatoes.)

Basil, 1 bunch (Store upright in a container with 1 in. of fresh water covering cut stems, like a bouquet of fresh flowers.)

Bell peppers, 3 red, 1 green, 1 yellow (Store in plastic bag in produce bin of refrigerator.)

Blueberries, 2 cups (Store in original container in refrigerator.)

Broccoli, 2 cups (about 1 lb. or 1 medium head)

Carrots, 1 lb. (Store in plastic bag in produce bin of refrigerator.)

Carrots, baby (Store in plastic bag in produce bin of refrigerator.)

Celery, 1 bunch (Store in plastic bag in produce bin of refrigerator.)

Corn, 3 ears (Store in plastic bag in produce bin of refrigerator.)

Cucumbers, 4 (Store in produce bin of refrigerator; do not put waxed produce or produce with treated peel in plastic bags.)

Field greens, 1 (1-lb) pkg. ready-washed (Store in plastic bag in produce bin of refrigerator.)

Fruits for fondue (optional)

Garlic, 1 head (Store in brown paper bag in pantry; or you can purchase 1 small jar minced garlic and store in refrigerator.)

Grapefruit, 1 (Store in plastic bag in produce bin of refrigerator.)

Grapes, 1 bunch (Store in plastic bag in produce bin of refrigerator.)

Green beans, 2 cups (Store in plastic bag in produce bin of refrigerator.)

Jicama, 1 small (Store in plastic bag in produce bin of refrigerator.)

Kale, 1 bunch (Store in plastic bag in produce bin of refrigerator.)

Lemons, 2 (Store in plastic bag in produce bin of refrigerator.)

Lettuce, 2 heads romaine (Store in plastic bag in produce bin of refrigerator.)

Mushrooms, 1 lb. (Store in original packaging or, if loose, store in a brown paper bag in the produce bin of refrigerator.)

Onions, 2 bunches green (Store in plastic bag in produce bin of refrigerator.)

Onions, 3 red (Store in brown paper bag in pantry, away from heat, light, and potatoes.)

Onions, 1 lb. yellow (Store in brown paper bag in pantry, away from heat, light, and potatoes.)

Oranges, 3 (Store in plastic bag in produce bin of refrigerator.)

Parsley, 1 bunch Italian (Store standing in a container with 1-in. of fresh water covering cut stems, like a bouquet of fresh flowers.)

Pears, 2 (Store in plastic bag in produce bin of refrigerator.)

Plums, 4

Potato, 1 baking (Store in paper bag, unrefrigerated.)

Potatoes, 1 lb. small red (Store in pantry, away from heat, light, onions, and bananas.)

Radishes (Store in plastic bag in produce bin of refrigerator.)

Rosemary, 1 small bunch (Store standing in a container with 1 in. of fresh water covering cut stems, like a bouquet of fresh flowers.)

Salsa, 1 pint fresh (Store in refrigerator.)

Spinach, 2 (lb.) pkgs. ready-washed (Store in plastic bag in produce bin of refrigerator.)

Strawberries, 3 cups (Store in original container in refrigerator.)

Sweet potato, 1 (Store in pantry, away from heat, light, onions, and bananas.)

Swiss chard, 4 leaves

Tangerine, 1

Tomatoes, 3 lbs. (Store in pantry, away from heat, light, potatoes, and bananas.)

Tomatoes, 1 pint cherry (Store in pantry, away from heat, light, potatoes, and bananas.)

Watermelon, 1 small (Store in plastic bag in produce bin of refrigerator.)

Zucchini, 1 (Store in plastic bag in produce bin of refrigerator.)

Phase 2 Shopping List

DAIRY

Buttermilk, 1 pint reduced-fat (Freeze unused portion in ice-cube tray.)

Cheese, 1 (8-oz.) pkg. cheddar, reduced-fat

Cheese, 1 (1-lb.) container cream cheese, fat-free, or reduced-fat (Neufchâtel)

Cheese, 1 (6-oz.) container cream cheese, reduced-fat, garlic-herb spread

Cheese, 1 (4-oz.) pkg. Monterey Jack reduced-fat

Cheese, 1 (8-oz.) pkg. mozzarella, reduced-fat, or part skim milk, grated

Cheese, 1 (8-oz.) container ricotta, fat-free, or part skim milk

Cheese, 1 oz. soy cheese, cheddar or other flavor

Cheese, string, reduced-fat

Cheese, 1 oz. Swiss, reduced-fat, low-sodium

Cottage cheese, 1 pint fat-free or low-fat

Egg substitute or egg replacement, 1 qt. cholesterol-free

Eggs, 6 (Store in coldest part of refrigerator in original packaging.)

Frozen yogurt, 1 cup fat-free

Ice cream, ½ cup vanilla

Margarine, 1 (1-lb.) tub trans fat–free, light margarine, or spread

Milk, 1 gallon fat-free plus ½ cup 1%

Pudding, 2 cups sugar-free

Tofu, 3 (12.3-oz.) pkgs. firm or extra-firm

Yogurt, 1 cup fat-free vanilla

Yogurt, 1 pint nonfat plain

Meats, Poultry, and Seafood

Beef, 1 lb. sirloin steak (Buy fresh and freeze, or buy frozen.)

Chicken, 4 lbs. boneless, skinless breasts (Buy fresh and freeze, or buy frozen.)

Cod, 3.5 lbs. fillets (Buy fresh and freeze, or buy frozen.)

Ham, 3 oz. lunch meat–style (Store in refrigerator.)

Pork, 1 lb. tenderloin (Buy fresh and freeze, or buy frozen.)

Red snapper, 1 lb. fillet (Buy fresh and freeze, or buy frozen.)

Salmon, 1½ lb. fillet (Buy fresh and freeze, or buy frozen.)

Turkey breast, 3 oz. lunch meat–style (Store in refrigerator.)

Turkey, 1 lb. ground (Buy fresh and freeze, or buy frozen.)

Fresh Produce

Apples, 3 (about 1 lb.)

Avocado, 1 (Store in pantry, away from heat, light, potatoes, and bananas.)

Banana, 1 (Store in pantry, away from heat, light, and tomatoes.)

Bell peppers, 4 green, 3 red, 2 yellow or another color (Store in plastic bag in produce bin of refrigerator.)

Blackberries, 1 cup (about 1 pint)

Blueberries, 2½ cups (Cover with dry paper towel and store in plastic bag in refrigerator.)

Broccoli, 2 cups (about 1 lb. or 1 medium head)

Cabbage, 1 head green; or you can purchase a 1 lb. pkg. shredded green cabbage (Store in plastic bag in produce bin of refrigerator.)

Cantaloupe, 1 (Store in refrigerator. Be sure to wash the outside of the melon and dry with a paper towel before cutting. After cutting, cover cut surface with plastic wrap, and then refrigerate.)

Carrots, 1 lb. (Store in plastic bag in produce bin of refrigerator.)

Carrots, baby (about 1 lb.)

Cauliflower, 1 cup (about ½ lb. or 1 very small head)

Celery, 1 bunch (Store in plastic bag in produce bin of refrigerator.)

Chiles: 3 serrano or jalapeño (Store in

plastic bag in produce bin of refrigerator.)

Chives (about 1 bunch) or substitute 1 bunch green onions

Cilantro, 1 bunch (Store standing in a container with 1 in. of fresh water covering cut stems, like a bouquet of fresh flowers.)

Corn, 1 ear

Cucumbers, 2 medium (Store in produce bin of refrigerator; do not put waxed produce in plastic bags.)

Eggplants, 2 (Store in produce bin of refrigerator; do not put waxed produce or produce with treated peel in plastic bags.)

Garlic, 2 heads (Store in brown paper bag; or you can purchase 1 small jar minced garlic and store in refrigerator.)

Ginger, 8 oz. (Store in plastic bag in produce bin of refrigerator.)

Grapefruit, 1 (Store in plastic bag in produce bin of refrigerator.)

Grapes, ½ cup (1 very small bunch)

Green beans, 1 cup (about ¼ lb.)

Jicama, 2 cups (about 1 lb. or 1 small)

Kiwi, 1 (Store in plastic bag in produce bin of refrigerator.)

Lemons, 2 (Store in plastic bag in produce bin of refrigerator.)

Lettuce, 2 heads romaine (Store in plastic bag in produce bin of refrigerator.)

Mint, 1 bunch (Store standing in a container with 1 in. of fresh water covering cut stems.)

Mushrooms, 2 lbs. presliced, if you like (Store in original packaging; if loose, store in a brown paper bag in produce bin of refrigerator.)

Mushrooms, 1 cup shiitake (You can use ½ cup dried shiitakes, and reconstitute them in ½ cup warm water for 10 minutes. Store in original packaging; if loose, store in a brown paper bag in produce bin of refrigerator.)

Nectarine, 1 (Store in plastic bag in produce bin of refrigerator.)

Onions, 2 bunches green (Store in plastic bag in produce bin of refrigerator.)

Onions, 2 red (Store in brown paper bag in pantry, away from heat, light, and potatoes.)

Onion: 1 lb. yellow (Store in brown paper bag in pantry, away from heat, light, and potatoes.)

Oranges, 3 (Store in plastic bag in produce bin of refrigerator.)

Parsley, 1 bunch Italian (Store standing in a container with 1 in. of fresh water covering cut stems, like a bouquet of fresh flowers.)

Peach, 1 (Store in plastic bag in produce bin of refrigerator.)

Pear, 1 (Store in plastic bag in produce bin of refrigerator.)

Plums, 2 (Store in plastic bag in produce bin of refrigerator.)

Spinach, 2 lbs. (Store in plastic bag in produce bin of refrigerator.)

Strawberries, 3 cups (Cover with dry paper towel and store in plastic bag in refrigerator.)

Tomatoes, 2 lbs. plum (Store in pantry, away from heat, light, and bananas.)

Yam, 1 large (Store in pantry, away from heat, light, and onions.)

Zucchini, 2 lbs. (Store in plastic bag in produce bin of refrigerator.)

Phase 3 Shopping List

Dairy

Cheese, 1 oz. reduced-fat cheddar

Cheese, 4 oz. reduced-fat feta

Cheese, ½ oz. provolone

Cheese, string, 4 servings reduced-fat

Cottage cheese, 1 pint

Egg substitute or egg replacement, 2 qt. cholesterol-free

Eggs, 6

Frozen yogurt, 1 pint vanilla

Half-and-half, 8 oz. fat-free

Milk, 1 gallon fat-free

Tofu, 1 (12.3-oz.) pkg. firm or extra-firm

Yogurt, 1 cup coffee-flavored (or other flavor)

Yogurt, 1 pint nonfat plain

Yogurt, 2 cups nonfat vanilla

Meat, Poultry, and Seafood

Beef, 2 lbs. rump roast (Buy fresh and freeze, or buy frozen.)

Beef, 2 lbs. top round steak (Buy fresh and freeze, or buy frozen.)

Chicken, 4 lbs. boneless, skinless breasts (Buy fresh and freeze, or buy frozen.)

Cod, 8 oz. fillets (Buy fresh and freeze, or buy frozen.)

Pork, 6 (5-oz.) chops

Shrimp, 1 lb.

Trout, 1½ lbs. fillets (Buy fresh and freeze, or buy frozen.)

Turkey, 1 lb. bacon, reduced-fat (Buy packaged and freeze.)

Turkey, 2 lb. breast, fresh (Buy fresh and freeze, or buy frozen.)

Turkey, 1 lb. ground (Buy fresh and freeze, or buy frozen.)

Vegetarian sausage, 1 small pkg. frozen, any flavor

Veggie burgers, 1 small pkg. frozen, any flavor

Fresh Produce

Apples, 7 (Store in plastic bag in produce bin of refrigerator.)

Asparagus, 1 lb. (Store in plastic bag in produce bin of refrigerator.)

Bananas, 4 (Store in pantry, away from heat, light, and tomatoes.)

Basil, 1 bunch (Store standing in a container with 1 in. of fresh water covering cut stems, like a bouquet of fresh flowers.)

Beets, 1 cup (Store in plastic bag in produce bin of refrigerator.)

Bell peppers, 2 green, 2 red (Store in plastic bag in produce bin of refrigerator.)

Blackberries, 1 pint, or another type of seeded berry, if you prefer (Cover with dry paper towel and store in plastic bag in produce bin of refrigerator.)

Broccoli, 2 lbs., or the ready-to-cook broccoli crowns, if you prefer (Store in plastic bag in produce bin of refrigerator.)

Cabbage, 1 head green, or you can purchase a 1 lb. pkg. shredded green cabbage (Store in plastic bag in produce bin of refrigerator.)

Cabbage, 1 small head purple (Store in plastic bag in produce bin of refrigerator.)

Carrots, 1 lb. (Store in plastic bag in produce bin of refrigerator.)

Cauliflower, ½ cup (about ½ lb. or 1 very small head)

Celery, 1 bunch (Store in plastic bag in produce bin of refrigerator.)

Chiles, 2 red (Store in plastic bag in produce bin of refrigerator.)

Cilantro, 1 bunch (Store standing in a container with 1-in. of fresh water covering cut stems, like a bouquet of fresh flowers.)

Cucumbers, 2 (Store in produce bin of refrigerator; do not put waxed produce in plastic bags.)

Eggplant, 1 small (Store in produce bin of refrigerator; do not put waxed produce or produce with treated peel in plastic bags.)

Garlic, 2 heads (Store in pantry, away from heat, light, potatoes, and bananas.)

Grapefruit, 1 (Store in plastic bag in produce bin of refrigerator.)

Grapes, 1 lb. green (Store in plastic bag in produce bin of refrigerator.)

Green beans, 1 cup (about ¼ lb.)

Honeydew melon: 1 small (store in refrigerator. Be sure to wash the outside of the melon and dry with a paper towel before cutting. After cutting, cover cut surface with plastic wrap, then refrigerate.)

Jalapeño pepper, 1 (Store in plastic bag in produce bin of refrigerator.)

Kale, 2 cups (about 1 bunch) (Store in plastic bag in produce bin of refrigerator.)

Kiwi, 1 (Store in plastic bag in produce bin of refrigerator.)

Lettuce, 3 heads romaine (Store in plastic bag in produce bin of refrigerator.)

Mushrooms, 1 lb. button (Store in original packaging, or if loose, store in a brown paper bag in produce bin of refrigerator.)

Onions, 1 bunch green (Store in plastic bag in produce bin of refrigerator.)

Onions, 3 red/purple (Store in pantry, away from heat, light, and potatoes.)

Onions, 2 lbs. yellow (Store in brown paper bag in pantry, away from heat, light, and potatoes.)

Oranges, 2 (Store in plastic bag in produce bin of refrigerator.)

Papaya, 2

Parsley, 1 bunch (Store standing in a container with 1 in. of fresh water covering cut stems, like a bouquet of fresh flowers.)

Peaches, 9 (Store in plastic bag in produce bin of refrigerator.)

Pear, 3

Pineapple, 1 (Store in plastic bag in produce bin of refrigerator.)

Potato, 1 baking (Store in brown paper bag in pantry away from heat, light, and onions.)

Potatoes, 2 russet (Store in brown paper bag in pantry, away from heat, light, and onions.)

Raspberries, 2 pints (Cover with dry paper towel and store in plastic bag in produce bin of refrigerator.)

Rutabagas, 2 (Store in plastic bag in produce bin of refrigerator.)

Snow peas, 8 oz. (Store in plastic bag in produce bin of refrigerator.)

Spinach, 12 cups (1 [10-oz.] pkg. prewashed)

Squash, 1 small butternut (Store in plastic bag in produce bin of refrigerator.)

Strawberries, 2 qt. (Cover with dry paper towel and store in plastic bag in produce bin of refrigerator.)

Tomatoes, 4 lbs. (Store in pantry, away from heat, light, and bananas.)

Watermelon, ½ small (Store in refrigerator. Be sure to wash the outside of the melon and dry with a paper towel before cutting. After cutting, cover cut surface with plastic wrap, then refrigerate.)

Yam, 1 (Store in brown paper bag in pantry away from heat, light, and onions.)

Zucchini, 2 lbs. (Store in plastic bag in produce bin of refrigerator.)

Vegetarian Meal Plan Shopping List—Days 1–5

PRODUCE

Apples, 2

Asparagus, 4 stalks

Bananas, 2

Bell peppers, 2 green, 4 red

Blueberries, 1½ cup

Bok choy, 1 bunch

Broccoli, 1 cup (about ½ lb. or 1 small head)

Carrots, 2

Celery, 1 bunch

Cilantro, 1 bunch

Cucumbers, 7

Eggplant, 2

Garlic, 2 heads or 1 small jar minced

Ginger, 1 (2-in.) piece

Grapes, 8 oz.

Green beans, 1 cup

Jalapeño peppers, 3

Kale, 2 bunches

Lemon, 1

Lettuce, 2 bunches romaine

Lime, 1

Mint, 2 sprigs fresh (You may use dried.)

Mushrooms, 2 cups sliced (about 8 oz.)

Mushrooms, 2 portobello

Onions, 5 cups chopped (about 2 lbs.) (You may buy prechopped.)

Onions, 1 bunch green

Onion, 1 red

Orange, 1

Parsley, 1 bunch Italian

Pear, 1

Pear, 1 Asian

Raisins, 2 one-pound boxes

Salad greens, 6 cups your favorite dark leafy greens

Spinach, 14 cups fresh (or 2 [8-oz.] pkgs. prewashed)

Snow peas, 1 cup

Squash, 2 acorn

Squash, 2 medium-size butternut

Swiss chard, 1 bunch

Strawberries, 1 pint

Tomatoes, 11 medium

Yam, 1 large

Zucchini, 4

FROZEN

Green beans, Italian (smallest package available)

Ice cream, 1 small carton reduced-fat chocolate (or your favorite flavor)

Spinach, 1 lb. frozen

Juices/Beverages/Alcohol for Cooking

Apple juice, ½ cup
Orange juice, 1 pint calcium-fortified
Sake, 2 Tbsp.

Spices

Arrowroot (or cornstarch, if unavailable)
Bay leaf
Black pepper
Cayenne pepper
Cinnamon
Cloves
Cream of tartar
Cumin
Dill weed
Garam masala (optional)
NutriFit Calypso Salt Free Spice Blend
NutriFit Lemon Garden Salt Free Spice Blend
NutriFit Mediterranean Salt Free Spice Blend
Red pepper flakes, crushed (optional)
Thyme
Turmeric

Canned Vegetables/Fruits/Prepared Foods

Artichoke hearts, 1 (8-oz.) jar marinated
Baby food prunes, 1 (2.5-oz.) container
Broth, 1 pint vegetable
Fruit cocktail in juice (or use fresh fruit instead)
Olives, 1 small can sliced black
Olives, 1 small jar green
Preserves, 1 small jar all-fruit strawberry

Salad dressing, 1 small bottle low-fat (less than 5 g fat/serving) or fat-free
Tomatoes, 1 (28-oz.) can
Tomato paste, 1 small can
Tomato salsa, 1 cup chunky
Water chestnuts, 1 can sliced

Condiments/Baking Goods

Balsamic vinegar
Baking powder
Baking soda
Brown sugar (smallest pkg.)
Canola oil
Canola oil cooking spray
Chocolate chips, 1 (12-oz.) pkg. semisweet
Cocoa powder, unsweetened
Cornstarch
Flour, 5 cups white unbleached all-purpose (about 2 lbs.)
Flour, 3 cups whole-wheat (about 1 lb.)
Hoisin sauce, 1 small jar
Honey, 1 small jar
Maple syrup
Mayonnaise, fat-free
Milk, 1 (12-oz.) can evaporated fat-free
Molasses, blackstrap
Mustard, at least 1 cup, dijon
Olive oil, extra-virgin
Olive oil spray, extra-virgin
Sesame oil (smallest bottle)
Soy sauce, 1 bottle reduced-sodium
Sugar, at least 5 cups (about 2 lbs.)
Sugar, powdered
Tamari, reduced-sodium
Tabasco sauce

Vanilla extract

Vinegar, 1 tsp. apple-cider (or other salad vinegar)

Vinegar, 1 small bottle red-wine

Vinegar, rice, unseasoned

Worcestershire sauce

GRAINS/CEREALS/SNACKS

Bran flakes, unsweetened

Bread, 1 (pkg. of 6) whole-wheat pita

Bread, 1 small loaf whole-wheat (You will need 2 slices; freeze the unused portion.)

Cereal, 1 small box shredded-wheat

Cereal, 1 small box whole-grain breakfast with at least 6 g dietary fiber and protein/serving

Chex Mix (smallest bag)

Crackers, 1 small box whole-grain animal

Crackers, 1 small box whole-grain graham

Millet, ½ cup

Noodles, 8 oz. udon and soba

Oats for oatmeal cereal, 1 cup instant or other

Pretzels, 1 cup whole-wheat

Quinoa, 2 cups

Rice, 3 cups brown

Tortillas, 1 dozen corn

Wheat germ

LEGUMES/NUTS/SEEDS/PROTEINS

Almonds (2-oz. pkg.)

Beans, 1 lb. black

Beans, 1 (15-oz.) can reduced-sodium garbanzo

Beans, ½ lb. pinto

Eggs, 5

Lentils, 4 oz.

Peanut butter, 1 jar reduced-fat, all-natural

Peanuts, 3 oz.

Pine nuts, 1 (2-oz.) pkg.

Pistachio nuts, 1 (2-oz.) pkg.

Pumpkin seeds, 1 (2-oz.) pkg.

Sesame seeds, 2 Tbsp.

Tofu, 2 (12.3-oz.) pkgs. extra-firm, reduced-fat

Soy nuts, ¾ cup roasted

Soy taco meat, 1½ oz.

Sunflower seed kernels, ½ cup

Walnuts, 1 (2-oz.) pkg.

DAIRY/DAIRY EQUIVALENT

Cheese, 1 cup reduced-fat cheddar, grated

Cheese, 1 (4-oz.) container fat-free cream cheese, or Neufchâtel light

Cheese, 1 cup part-skim milk mozzarella, grated

Cheese, string, 1 reduced-fat

Cottage cheese, 1 pint fat-free

Egg substitute, 1 qt. fat-free

Margarine or spread, 1 small carton trans fat–free, light

Milk, 1 gallon fat-free

Soy cheese, 2 oz.

Yogurt, 1 cup nonfat vanilla

Vegetarian Meal Plan Shopping List—Days 6–15

FRESH PRODUCE

Apples, 4

Bananas, 5

Basil, 1 bunch

Bell peppers, 5 red, 3 green, and 1 any color, large

Blueberries, 1 pint

Broccoli flowerets, 1 lb.

Cabbage, 1 small pkg. (or 1 small wedge) purple, shredded

Cantaloupe, 1

Carrots, 1 lb.

Carrots, 1 (1-lb.) pkg. baby

Cauliflower, 1 cup (about ¼ lb.)

Celery, 1 bunch

Chives, 1 bunch

Cilantro, 1 bunch

Cucumber, 1

Dill weed, 1 bunch

Eggplant, 2 large

Fennel bulb, 1

Garlic, at least 3 heads fresh; or 1 jar chopped garlic

Ginger, 1 (2-in.) piece fresh

Grapefruit, 1

Grapes, ½ cup (about ¼ lb.)

Green beans, 3 cups (about 1 lb.)

Jalapeño pepper, 1

Jicama, 1 (about 1 lb., at least 2 cups sliced into sticks)

Leek, 1

Lemons, 5

Lettuce, 1 head red leaf

Lettuce, 1 head romaine

Limes, 2

Melon, 1 honeydew

Mint, 1 bunch

Mushrooms, 2 lbs.

Nectarine, 1

Onions, 2 bunches green

Onion, 5 red

Onions, 5–6 (about 2 lbs.), yellow or white

Oranges, 4

Parsley, 1 bunch Italian

Peach, 1

Pineapple, 2 cups cut up

Potatoes, 1 lb. small red

Potatoes, 1 lb. russet

Spinach, 2 bunches fresh or 1 (1-lb.) pkg. plus 1 ten-oz. pkg.

Sprouts, 1 pint alfalfa

Sprouts, 1 lb. bean

Squash, 1 acorn

Squash, 1 cup (about ¼ lb.) summer

Summer strawberries, 1 pint

Swiss chard, 1 bunch red or green

Tomatoes, 3 lbs. plus 8 whole

Tomatoes, 1 pint cherry

Tomatoes, 4 (about 1 lb.) Italian plum

Yam or sweet potato, 1

Zucchini, 3 (about ¾ lb.)

FROZEN FOODS

Apple-juice concentrate, 1 (6-oz.) can frozen

Blueberries, 1 cup frozen

Cherries, 1 cup frozen, pitted

Corn, 1 lb. frozen

Frozen yogurt, 1 cup fat-free vanilla

Green peas, 1 lb. frozen

Spinach, 3 lbs. frozen chopped

Strawberries, 1 cup frozen

Juices, Beverages, Alcohol for Cooking

Apple juice, 1 (48-oz.) bottle

Orange juice, 1 qt. (preferably calcium-fortified)

Prune juice, 2 cups

White wine, 1 small bottle alcoholic or nonalcoholic (for cooking)

V8 juice, 2 cups reduced-sodium

Canned Vegetables, Fruit (Canned and Dried), Prepared Foods

Artichoke hearts, 1 (8-oz.) can water-packed (if available)

Apricot halves, 1 (8-oz.) can juice-packed (if available)

Broth, 5 qts. vegetable (choose a brand that is lower in sodium)

Chiles, 1 (4-oz.) can green, diced

Currants, 1 small box (or you may use raisins)

Dates, 2 Tbsp. unsweetened

Dried figs, 1 lb.

Dried fruit, 2½ cups mixed

Enchilada sauce, 1 (8-oz.) can

Marinara sauce, 5 cups

Pineapple slices, 1 (8-oz.) can juice-packed (if available)

Pudding, 1 pkg. instant chocolate, or 1 small container prepared chocolate pudding

Raisins, 1 lb.

Raisins, golden or black, 1 (8-oz. or smaller) box

Tomato salsa, 1 pint fresh

Tomatoes, 4 (28-oz.) cans, reduced-sodium Italian plum (or whole tomatoes)

Grains, Cereals, Snacks

Bagels, 2 whole-wheat

Barley, 1 bag (about 1 lb.) pearl

Biscotti, 1

Bread, 1 loaf whole-wheat

Bread, 6 slices whole-wheat cinnamon

Bread, whole-wheat pita

Bread, round (optional for serving dip)

Breadcrumbs, 1 cup whole-wheat (or make your own by processing 3 slices whole-wheat bread in a food processor)

Couscous, 2 cups whole-wheat (about 1 lb.)

Crackers, graham

Crackers, whole grain

English muffin, 1 whole-wheat

Lavosh, 1 pkg. (fresh, whole-wheat) or lavosh crackers

Noodles, lasagna

Oats, 2½ cups quick-cooking rolled (about 1 lb.)

Pasta, 1 lb. dry whole-wheat

Pretzels, peanut-butter filled

Pretzels, whole-grain

Rice, 2 lbs. brown (or at least 7 cups dry measure)

Soy nuts, 20 oz.

Tortillas, 1 (8-oz.) pkg. corn

Tortillas, at least 9 whole-wheat (preferably fat-free, or lower in fat)

Vegetarian "chicken" nuggets (about ½ lb.)

Wheat bran, 1 small pkg.

Legumes, Nuts, Seeds, Proteins

Almonds, 1 (4-oz. or smaller) pkg. slivered

Beans, 1 lb. dried black (at least 5 cups)

Beans, 1 can cannellini

Beans, 2 cans reduced-sodium garbanzo

Beans, 1 can vegetarian refried

Beans, 1 (1 lb.) can white

Black-eyed peas, 8 oz. dried

Egg substitute, liquid, 2 (32-oz.) cartons

Egg whites, 1 (32-oz.) carton (or 1 dozen extra eggs for separating)

Eggs, 6

Green split peas, 1 small pkg. dried

Ground-meat alternative, 12 oz.

Hummus, 1 small container

Lentils, ½ cup (or small pkg.) dried

Lentils, 8 oz. red

Peanut butter, 1 jar reduced-fat, all-natural

Peanuts, 1 small pkg.

Tofu, 7 (12.3-oz. or larger) pkgs.

Sesame seeds, 1 small jar (or tin)

Soybeans (or you may use frozen shelled edamame), 1 (1 lb.) pkg.

Walnut halves, 8 oz.

DAIRY, DAIRY EQUIVALENTS

Buttermilk, 1 pint reduced-fat

Cheese, 3 (8-oz.) pkgs. fat-free cream cheese (if available) or Neufchâtel light cream cheese

Cheese, 1 (4-oz.) pkg. cream cheese lite garlic-herb, soft-spread

Cheese, 1-lb. reduced-fat, shredded cheddar

Cheese, 1 (6-oz.) pkg. reduced-fat feta

Cheese, 1 cup (4-oz.) reduced-fat, shredded Monterey Jack

Cheese, 1 (8-oz.) pkg. reduced-fat (part-skim milk, or fat-free) mozzarella

Cheese, 1 container reduced-fat or fat-free grated Parmesan

Cheese, 1 qt. reduced-fat (part-skim milk, or fat-free) ricotta

Cottage cheese, 1 qt. plus 1 pint fat-free

Margarine, 1 lb. trans fat–free

Milk, 2 (12-oz.) cans evaporated fat-free

Milk, 1 qt. fat-free

Milk, 1 (8-oz.) container 1%

Milk, 12 cups fat-free vanilla soy

Sour cream, 1½ cups fat-free

Yogurt, 1½ cups fat-free plain

Yogurt, 2½ cups fat-free fruit-flavored

Yogurt, 1 cup fat-free vanilla

body mass index chart

BMI (kg/m2)	19	20	21	22	23	24	25	26	27	28	29	30	35	40
Height (in.)							Weight (lbs.)							
58	91	96	100	105	110	115	119	124	129	134	138	143	167	191
59	94	99	104	109	114	119	124	128	133	138	143	148	173	198
60	97	102	107	112	118	123	128	133	138	143	148	153	179	204
61	100	106	111	116	122	127	132	137	143	148	153	158	185	211
62	104	109	115	120	126	131	136	142	147	153	158	164	191	218
63	107	113	118	124	130	135	141	146	152	158	163	169	197	225
64	110	116	122	128	134	140	145	151	157	163	169	174	204	232
65	114	120	126	132	138	144	150	156	162	168	174	180	210	240
66	118	124	130	136	142	148	155	161	167	173	179	186	216	247
67	121	127	134	140	146	153	159	166	172	178	185	191	223	255
68	125	131	138	144	151	158	164	171	177	184	190	197	230	262
69	128	135	142	149	155	162	169	176	182	189	196	203	236	270
70	132	139	146	153	160	167	174	181	188	195	202	207	243	278
71	136	143	150	157	165	172	179	186	193	200	208	215	250	286
72	140	147	154	162	169	177	184	191	199	206	213	221	258	294
73	144	151	159	166	174	182	189	197	204	212	219	227	265	302
74	148	155	163	171	179	186	194	202	210	218	225	233	272	311
75	152	160	168	176	184	192	200	208	216	224	232	240	279	319
76	156	164	172	180	189	197	205	213	221	230	238	246	287	328

See page 153 for an interpretation of this BMI chart.

recipe index

general index

body after baby

body after baby

A SIMPLE, HEALTHY PLAN TO LOSE YOUR BABY WEIGHT FAST

Jackie Keller

AVERY
A MEMBER OF
PENGUIN GROUP (USA) INC.
NEW YORK

AVERY

Published by the Penguin Group

Penguin Group (USA) Inc., 375 Hudson Street, New York, New York 10014, USA • Penguin Group (Canada), 90 Eglinton Avenue East, Suite 700, Toronto, Ontario M4P 2Y3, Canada (a division of Pearson Penguin Canada Inc.) • Penguin Books Ltd, 80 Strand, London WC2R 0RL, England • Penguin Ireland, 25 St Stephen's Green, Dublin 2, Ireland (a division of Penguin Books Ltd) • Penguin Group (Australia), 250 Camberwell Road, Camberwell, Victoria 3124, Australia (a division of Pearson Australia Group Pty Ltd) • Penguin Books India Pvt Ltd, 11 Community Centre, Panchsheel Park, New Delhi—110 017, India • Penguin Group (NZ), 67 Apollo Drive, Rosedale, North Shore 0745, Auckland, New Zealand (a division of Pearson New Zealand Ltd) • Penguin Books (South Africa) (Pty) Ltd, 24 Sturdee Avenue, Rosebank, Johannesburg 2196, South Africa

Penguin Books Ltd, Registered Offices: 80 Strand, London WC2R 0RL, England

First trade paperback edition 2007
Copyright © 2006 by Jackie Keller
Illustrations by Peter Young
All rights reserved. No part of this book may be reproduced, scanned, or distributed in any printed or electronic form without permission. Please do not participate in or encourage piracy of copyrighted materials in violation of the author's rights. Purchase only authorized editions. Published simultaneously in Canada

Most Avery books are available at special quantity discounts for bulk purchase for sales promotions, premiums, fund-raising, and educational needs. Special books or book excerpts also can be created to fit specific needs. For details, write Penguin Group (USA) Inc. Special Markets, 375 Hudson Street, New York, NY 10014.

The Library of Congress catalogued the hardcover edition as follows:

Keller, Jackie.
Body after baby: a simple plan to lose your baby weight fast/Jackie Keller.
p.   cm.
Includes index.
ISBN 1-58333-251-0
1. Postnatal care.   2. Puerperium—Nutritional aspects.   3. Weight loss.   4. Exercise for women.   5. Physical fitness for women.   6. Mothers—Health and hygiene.   I. Title.
RG831.K45   2006   2006042745
618.6—dc22

ISBN 978-1-58333-280-1 (paperback edition)

Printed in the United States of America
10 9 8 7 6 5 4 3 2 1

BOOK DESIGN BY TANYA MAIBORODA

The recipes contained in this book are to be followed exactly as written. The publisher is not responsible for your specific health or allergy needs that may require medical supervision. The publisher is not responsible for any adverse reactions to the recipes contained in this book.

Neither the publisher nor the author is engaged in rendering professional advice or services to the individual reader. The ideas, procedures, and suggestions contained in this book are not intended as a substitute for consulting with your physician. All matters regarding your health require medical supervision. Neither the author nor the publisher shall be liable or responsible for any loss or damage allegedly arising from any information or suggestion in this book.

While the author has made every effort to provide accurate telephone numbers and Internet addresses at the time of publication, neither the publisher nor the author assumes any responsibility for errors, or for changes that occur after publication. Further, the publisher does not have any control over and does not assume any responsibility for author or third-party websites or their content.

Penguin Group (USA) is not associated with NutriFit or the Body After Baby program.